10
STEPS
TO CHANGE

How to
Manage Your

ECO-
ANXIETY

WRITTEN BY
ANOUCHKA GROSE

ILLUSTRATED BY
LAURIANE BOHÉMIER

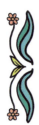

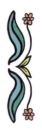

FOR ALL PEOPLE EVERYWHERE WHO ARE
WORKING TO PROTECT THE PLANET - A.G.

FOR ANYONE WHO WANTS TO CHANGE THE
WORLD, ONE ACT OF KINDNESS AT A TIME - L.B.

MAGIC CAT
PUBLISHING

10 Steps to Change: How to Manage Your Eco-Anxiety © 2023 Lucky Cat
Publishing Ltd
Text © 2023 Anouchka Grose
Illustrations by Lauriane Bohémier
First Published in 2023 by Magic Cat Publishing, an imprint of Lucky Cat
Publishing Ltd, Unit 2 Empress Works, 24 Grove Passage, London E2 9FQ, UK

A catalogue record for this book is available from the British Library.

ISBN 978-1-913520-76-2

The illustrations were created digitally
Set in Cherry, Wisely and Wilden

Published by Rachel Williams and Jenny Broom
Designed by Maisy Ruffels
Edited by Helen Brown

Printed in Slovenia

9 8 7 6 5 4 3 2 1

MIX
Paper from
responsible sources
FSC® C126477

☮ Contents ☮

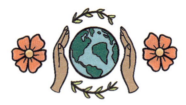

Welcome to this book about eco-anxiety.

I'm Anouchka and I'm a psychoanalyst, which means I spend all day listening to people speak about their thoughts and feelings - especially the things that make them sad, angry or scared. I work with young people, old people and everyone in the middle. And, thanks to the internet, I work with people from all over the world. One of the things I hear more and more is that people are scared about the future of the planet. They say things like:

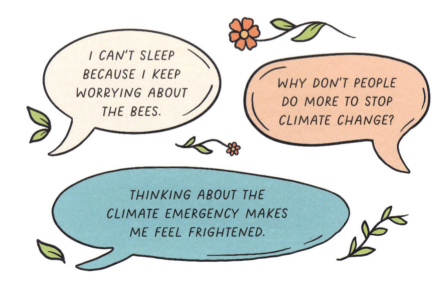

I CAN'T SLEEP BECAUSE I KEEP WORRYING ABOUT THE BEES.

WHY DON'T PEOPLE DO MORE TO STOP CLIMATE CHANGE?

THINKING ABOUT THE CLIMATE EMERGENCY MAKES ME FEEL FRIGHTENED.

The last thing these people want to hear is, "Don't worry, it'll be fine." Sometimes their friends and family say this to them, and it makes them go, "Aaaaarrrrggghh!" or even, "If everyone thought like that, we'd all be doomed!"

When people are worried about climate change, they need other people to take their fears seriously. In a sense, the more of us who are worried about it the better. But we also need to feel OK. We need to sleep, eat and to remember that life on earth is an ongoing miracle. That's why we want to preserve it.

This book is a collection of all the things I've learned from working with people with eco-anxiety. It's a book that aims to care for the people most ready to help save the planet. I hope that reading it can help you to feel better. While I can't make the problem go away, I can tell you what scientists, activists and people living in countries on the frontline of climate change have said about the things that have helped them. I can also tell you what helps me. There will be ten steps, and a toolkit at the end of each step that will give you ways to handle your thoughts and feelings.

The main thing you need to remember is that you're not alone. It's really important to talk about your fears and also to know that there are plenty of things you can do to help the planet.

In fact, if you have eco-anxiety then congratulations! You're already halfway to being part of a solution...

What is eco-anxiety?

Eco-anxiety is extreme worry about current and future harm to the environment, and what I want you to understand about it is that it isn't a mental illness. **In fact, it's the exact opposite of an illness - it's a reasonable response to a real problem.** Some environmentalists aren't sure about the term 'eco-anxiety' because it makes it sound like a clinical anxiety disorder - for example 'social anxiety' (fear of social situations) or 'separation anxiety' (fear of losing the people you care about).

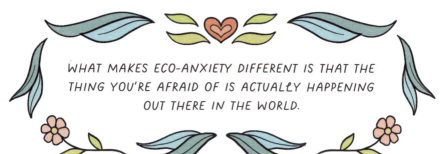

WHAT MAKES ECO-ANXIETY DIFFERENT IS THAT THE THING YOU'RE AFRAID OF IS ACTUALLY HAPPENING OUT THERE IN THE WORLD.

Because of this, some environmentalists prefer to use words, like 'climate grief', 'eco-trauma', 'green guilt' or 'climate change distress'. The advantage of these terms is that they don't make you sound like you're worrying unnecessarily. Plus, they make space for some of the other feelings you might be experiencing, like sadness, anger, shame, or even shutting down altogether.

Whatever term you prefer to use, if you're feeling any emotion right now, from anger to worry, I want you to know that you're far from alone. All of these feelings are absolutely normal, and we'll be exploring ways to manage them in the pages to come.

Who suffers from eco-anxiety?

Absolutely anyone and everyone! Young, old, rich, poor, city-dwellers, farmers, whoever. You could even argue that some people suffer from it without realising. Maybe they're too busy working out how to feed their families to let themselves think about it. Or perhaps they're pretending it isn't happening. In any case, it's harder and harder not to notice that our planet is at risk, even if you try to push it to the back of your mind.

Eco-anxiety isn't a new thing either. People have been speaking about it since the 1970s, when scientists and activists began warning people about the damage that was being done to the planet by fossil fuels, like coal and oil. Back then, climate change still seemed a long way off and scientists and activists often felt like they weren't being listened to. To make it worse, some politicians and business owners wrote them off as a bunch of foolish 'tree-huggers' (an epithet applied to someone who is very interested in protecting the environment). Now with hindsight we can probably agree that it was those politicians and business owners who were the foolish ones!

Today more and more people are experiencing these feelings as we hear about the real effects of climate change in the news. You may see it on the television, on social media, or in magazines and newspapers. Some older people feel terrible for not having acted sooner, and younger people are often frightened about the future. **What is clear is that we're all in it together.**

Is eco-anxiety normal?

Yes, eco-anxiety is normal. However, not everyone's experience of eco-anxiety is the same. All of us are different, so we register the same ideas and events in different ways. Then there's the fact that climate change is more noticeable in very hot and very cold climates. While in the Global North people might be worried about the future, for people in other parts of the world it's already happening. For example, people who live in Greenland and the Philippines are at opposite ends of the climate spectrum. Both countries are experiencing problems caused by extreme weather – either melting ice or storms.

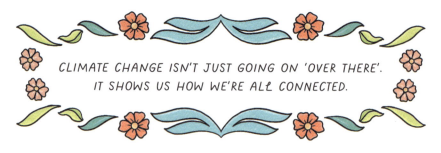

CLIMATE CHANGE ISN'T JUST GOING ON 'OVER THERE'. IT SHOWS US HOW WE'RE ALL CONNECTED.

The most important thing we can do is to look after ourselves, each other and the planet. It's vital to remember to do all three. If we don't take care of ourselves, we won't be able to take care of anything else. **So, the first step towards starting to deal with your eco-anxiety is to remember that it's OK to give yourself a break.** Some people like to sit still and take a deep breath. Others like to escape into a book or film. Maybe you love to run around, dance, sing, draw or make silly jokes. If it makes you feel better, do it! And I'm not just patronising you because you're a child – it's what marine biologists and eco-justice lawyers do… and psychotherapists like me, too!

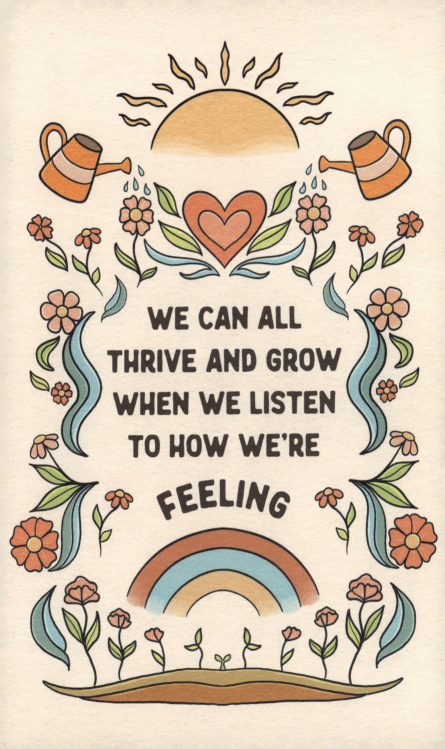

WE CAN ALL THRIVE AND GROW WHEN WE LISTEN TO HOW WE'RE FEELING

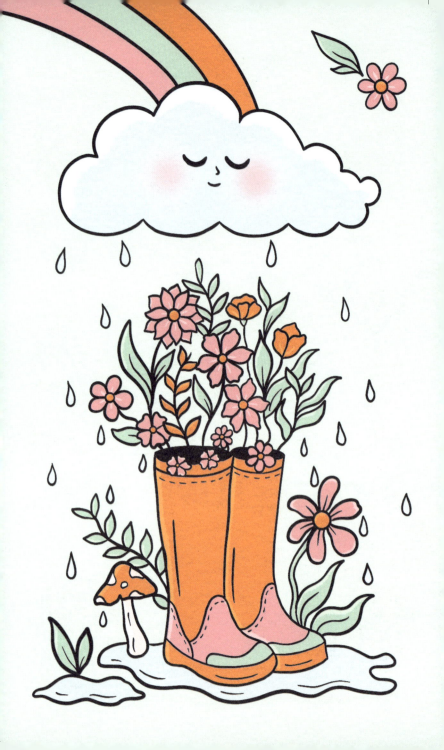

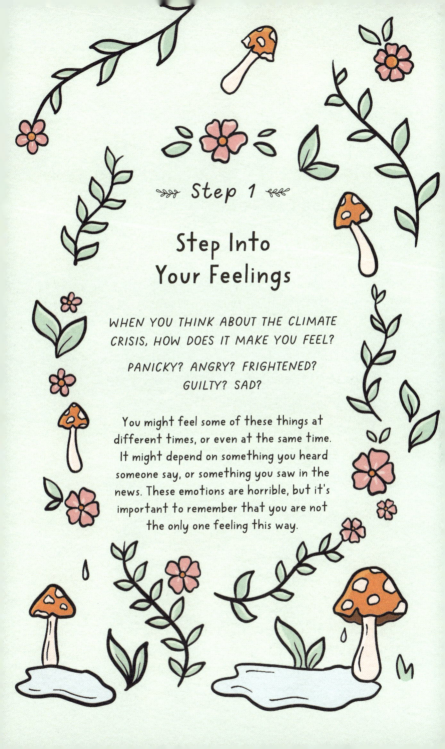

Step Into Your Feelings

WHEN YOU THINK ABOUT THE CLIMATE CRISIS, HOW DOES IT MAKE YOU FEEL?

PANICKY? ANGRY? FRIGHTENED? GUILTY? SAD?

You might feel some of these things at different times, or even at the same time. It might depend on something you heard someone say, or something you saw in the news. These emotions are horrible, but it's important to remember that you are not the only one feeling this way.

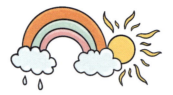

Sometimes it can be hard to tell what a feeling even is.

Is it a thought? A sensation? Or something in between? Sometimes our feelings are triggered by events out in the world, and sometimes they suddenly explode from somewhere deep inside us. One thing's for sure, they can be very hard to control. And eco-anxiety can be awful because it can feel like it will go on forever.

Mental signs of eco-anxiety include:

OUT OF CONTROL THOUGHTS

A SENSE OF DOOM

BRAIN FOG

GETTING CAUGHT UP IN THE FUTURE AND FORGETTING ABOUT THE PRESENT

Physical signs of eco-anxiety include:

FEELING SICK OR DIZZY

BREATHLESSNESS

A RACING HEART

HEADACHES

GOING CLAMMY ALL OVER

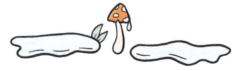

For most people, feelings of eco-anxiety come and go, only lasting a short time. This is because the human body isn't designed to exist in a constant state of emergency.

The other tricky thing about feelings is that it can be difficult to separate them all out. You might start by feeling sad, then angry, then you might feel guilty about your anger and then anxious about how sad, angry and guilty you feel. By the time someone asks you what's wrong, it's all such a mess in your head that you don't even know what to say, so you just say, "Hmph!" or sometimes you say nothing at all.

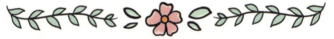

IT'S IMPORTANT TO REMEMBER THAT WHATEVER FEELINGS YOU'RE HAVING - EVEN IF THEY'RE NOT NICE TO FEEL - ARE OK.

The interesting bit is knowing what to do next. It can sometimes feel as though feelings aren't allowed. As soon as you show that you are upset, people either try to cheer you up, or tell you to stop being silly. But feelings aren't silly at all - they are often very clever.

Our feelings of eco-anxiety are reminding us that something is wrong. Some people deal with this by stamping their feelings out and refusing to acknowledge what's happening. Others might tell themselves it's all being solved - the politicians are working to fix it and, if that fails, technology will rescue us. Ignoring our feelings can often feel like the best solution to stop the pain we feel. It can feel like the only solution, and the relief we believe we'll feel by running away is very tempting. . . **But what if we listened to and engaged with our difficult feelings?**

In the same way that people from the same family or friendship group have very different ways of dealing with the same thing, everyone has their own ways of dealing with the climate crisis. Arguments can happen when people don't understand each other's ideas, feelings and reactions. Sometimes it's helpful to remember that other people's coping mechanisms might be different from yours. If other people seem to be in denial, that's just their way of dealing with it. But it doesn't have to be yours. If you suffer from eco-anxiety, it's because your mind isn't letting you run away from the problem.

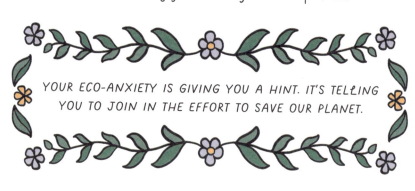

YOUR ECO-ANXIETY IS GIVING YOU A HINT. IT'S TELLING YOU TO JOIN IN THE EFFORT TO SAVE OUR PLANET.

It's important to know that your feelings about the climate crisis are legitimate. What's more, they have the potential to help you become part of the solution. Don't be hard on yourself. You should be proud of your feelings. They show that you are a well-informed, empathic person who cares about the state of the world. We don't want to get rid of your eco-anxiety, but to help you think of it instead as eco-compassion, eco-understanding, eco-action and eco-determination. It's a small switch from eco-worrier to eco-warrior - but you have to be worried in the first place to make it!

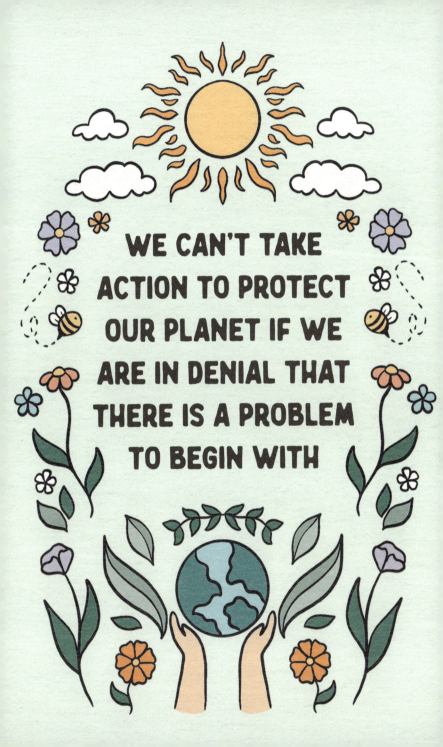

WE CAN'T TAKE
ACTION TO PROTECT
OUR PLANET IF WE
ARE IN DENIAL THAT
THERE IS A PROBLEM
TO BEGIN WITH

Self-care practices to ease your eco-anxiety

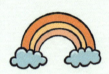

FOCUS ON THINGS THAT BRING YOU JOY

While it might be true to say that eco-anxiety is helpful for triggering action, it's also true that a love of life is a great motivator when it comes to preserving our world. So make time for the things you love - it'll make you a more effective eco-ally.

TALK TO SOMEONE YOU TRUST

It's awful to deal with bad feelings alone. Speak to someone you feel comfortable with and who will give you time to express your thoughts. Maybe choose a quiet moment, or tell them in advance that you need to have a proper chat about something that's upsetting you.

BE KIND TO YOURSELF

You don't have to be Greta Thunberg to make a difference. Even she probably doesn't feel like 'Greta Thunberg' all the time! Nobody's perfect, and the fact that you're worried at all shows you are the beginning of your journey towards becoming the best eco-ally you can be.

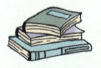

LEARN MORE ABOUT CLIMATE CHANGE

Learn about the things you can do to make difference, however big or small. We can often alleviate a fear of the unknown by educating ourselves about the situation in question. Knowledge is power, after all.

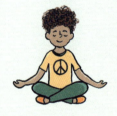

LISTEN TO YOUR BODY

Next time you watch the news and feel your heart speed up or your palms start sweating, check in with yourself and say, "Thank you, body, for reminding me how precious the world is. Please trust that I am doing what I can for now."

How to accept and value your feelings

1 VALIDATE YOUR ECO-ANXIETY

Whenever you feel eco-anxiety kick in, whether it's mental or physical, remind yourself that's it's a perfectly rational response to a real problem. Your eco-anxiety is a sign that your ideas and emotions are in tune.

2 REJECT DENIAL

You can't unknow what you already know. Once you've acknowledged that there's a problem, the only way is forwards. Denial might seem to work well for some people, but for those of us with eco-anxiety, it isn't really an option... and that's OK!

3 USE YOUR FEELINGS TO SPARK ACTION

Validating your feelings is the first step, and taking action is the second. Without action all the validation in the world could seem a little empty. Of course, you don't have to act straight away and maybe you're doing quite a bit already. Rather than piling on more pressure, you could remind yourself of the actions you're already taking.

4 FOSTER DETERMINATION

If you set yourself a realistic goal, like 'to live as responsibly and sustainably as possible', then you will increase your chances of achieving it. Make sure you forgive the odd deviation or slip up. It's not possible to be eco-perfect!

5 BE TOLERANT OF OTHERS

It's easy to get annoyed at people who have a bit of catching up to do with regard to the climate crisis. Belittling someone for having a different opinion to yours won't convince them to change their mind, but a thoughtful discussion might.

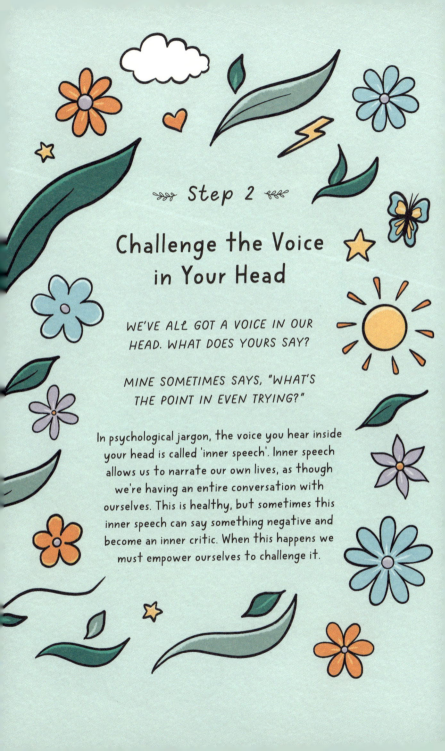

≫≫≫ Step 2 ≪≪≪

Challenge the Voice in Your Head

WE'VE ALL GOT A VOICE IN OUR HEAD. WHAT DOES YOURS SAY?

MINE SOMETIMES SAYS, "WHAT'S THE POINT IN EVEN TRYING?"

In psychological jargon, the voice you hear inside your head is called 'inner speech'. Inner speech allows us to narrate our own lives, as though we're having an entire conversation with ourselves. This is healthy, but sometimes this inner speech can say something negative and become an inner critic. When this happens we must empower ourselves to challenge it.

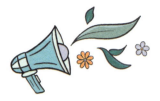

Whose voice is it anyway?

The strange thing about the voices in our heads is that it can be hard to say exactly whether they come from inside us or outside us. On the one hand, you could say they are our thoughts and no one else's. But who taught us how to think? The world bombards us with ideas and opinions and we gravitate towards some and steer clear of others. Still, our ideas and opinions can change. If the people around us don't seem bothered about climate change, it can be easy to treat some of their opinions as if they were our own. Sometimes we can even find ourselves having a private argument in our own head! Maybe it goes something like this:

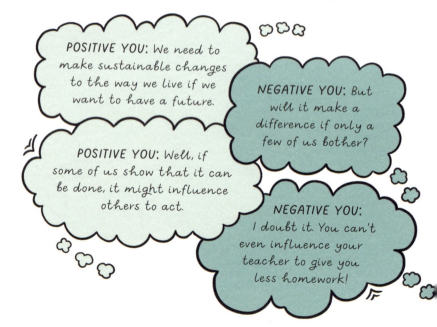

POSITIVE YOU: We need to make sustainable changes to the way we live if we want to have a future.

NEGATIVE YOU: But will it make a difference if only a few of us bother?

POSITIVE YOU: Well, if some of us show that it can be done, it might influence others to act.

NEGATIVE YOU: I doubt it. You can't even influence your teacher to give you less homework!

Psychologists call these confusing voices 'cognitive dissonance'. Cognitive dissonance means having two or more opposing ideas at the same time. Maybe you think it's pointless to eat a plant-based diet because hardly anyone else that you know does. But you also feel terrible every time you eat a beef burger. Or you've been told that recycling isn't going to save the world, but you can't bear to see a bin full of old food, paper, plastic and metal all mixed together.

One irritating feature of these conflicting voices is that it can be hard to tell which one's the 'real you'. Do you sincerely care about the planet but have a tendency to undermine your good intentions with self-destructive thoughts? Or is the real truth that you don't really want to have to go to a lot of effort to change your lifestyle as the effects of climate change don't impact you every day? For many of us, it tends to be a bit of both. We really do want what's best for the world, but we also know that we can sometimes be selfish or careless.

A certain amount of cognitive dissonance is inevitable - only a robot could be programmed to have perfectly consistent ideas! The rest of us have to accept a bit of psychological confusion. In fact, it's a sign that we are capable of complex thinking - it's good to be able to see both sides of an argument.

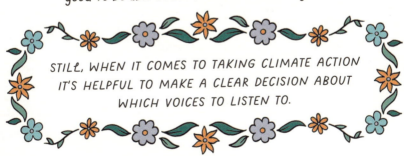

STILL, WHEN IT COMES TO TAKING CLIMATE ACTION IT'S HELPFUL TO MAKE A CLEAR DECISION ABOUT WHICH VOICES TO LISTEN TO.

You may not remember this but in 2019 Greta Thunberg told an American Congressional Hearing, "I don't want you to listen to me. I want you to listen to the scientists." This is a helpful way of thinking about who to listen to when we think about the climate crisis. There's no denying that scientists enjoy a good argument, but when it comes to climate change there is no debate. Scientists across the board agree that we need to act to reduce our carbon footprint - the total amount of greenhouse gases (including carbon dioxide and methane) that are generated by our actions. Every step we take in this direction is worthwhile. So, if a voice in your head is telling you it's all pointless, you should tell that voice to be quiet.

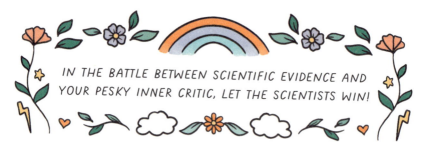

IN THE BATTLE BETWEEN SCIENTIFIC EVIDENCE AND YOUR PESKY INNER CRITIC, LET THE SCIENTISTS WIN!

Instead remind the voice that it's science that has helped us to understand the problem and offers us the methods to solve it. Science drives action and Greta Thunberg once famously said, "No one is too small to make a difference." I think we should definitely all listen to that! This doesn't mean we have to get super-stressed thinking of every possible thing we can do. It just means we should do something. If all of us make little differences today, it will make a massive difference to tomorrow.

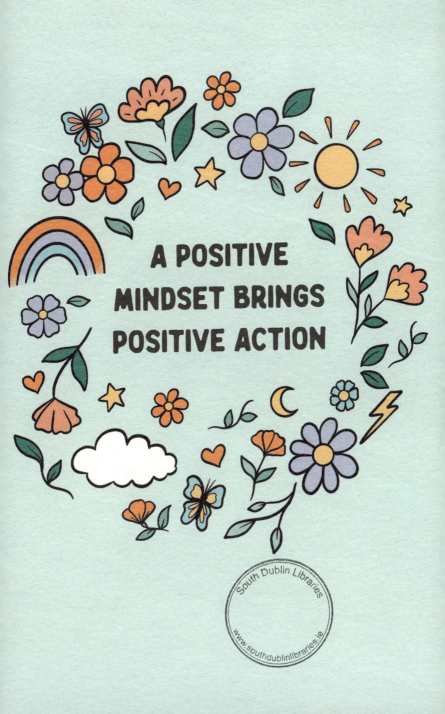

A POSITIVE
MINDSET BRINGS
POSITIVE ACTION

How to talk nicely to your inner critic

If you find yourself over-thinking, or getting into private arguments, don't worry: it's just a sign that your brain is taking all sorts of information into account. But instead of getting into an argument with your inner critic, you could try having a polite word. Here's an example:

POSITIVE YOU: Let's turn the thermostat down by one degree.

NEGATIVE YOU: What will that do to help anything?

POSITIVE YOU: It's just one small change among many. I will also be buying my clothes from second-hand shops and will stop eating meat for the entire month of January.

NEGATIVE YOU: Christmas followed by a month of lentils. Ugh!

POSITIVE YOU: I seem to remember you rather liking those veggie sausages. And tomato sauce is vegan every month of the year.

NEGATIVE YOU: If you say so.

POSITIVE YOU: I do, and what I say goes because we have a planet to save. I'm afraid I'm not listening to you anymore - I'm listening to the scientists.

Ways to ease your inner critic

REMIND YOURSELF YOU'RE NOT A ROBOT

Being human is very complicated and we can't always control the thoughts that run through our heads. You can only try your best.

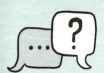

ASK QUESTIONS

Ask where that negative thought came from. Is it like something you heard on the radio? Or in the playground? Just because you thought it, it doesn't mean you have to keep thinking it. Perhaps it belongs to someone else anyhow.

RESPECT YOUR NEGATIVE VOICES

Negative voices are proof that your brain is hard at work. Don't feel bad about your own selfish, angry or defeatist thoughts – your mind is just sifting through the evidence. Confusion is very often a sign of intelligence.

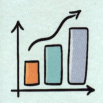

LET SCIENCE GIVE YOU HOPE

The evidence tells us that the climate scientists are right, and the scientists are telling us not to give up hope. The science is very clear – there are still lots of things we can do. So let's do them!

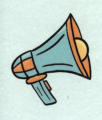

BE KIND TO YOUR NEGATIVE SELF

Just because your inner voices don't always agree, you don't need to become a human battlefield. Maybe your negative voices are just there for you to practice on. If you become good at talking them down nicely you will soon be ready to persuade real-life climate defeatists to start being more sensible!

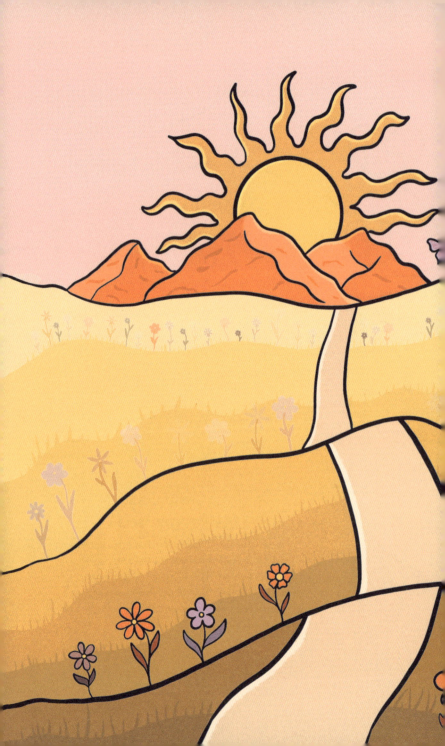

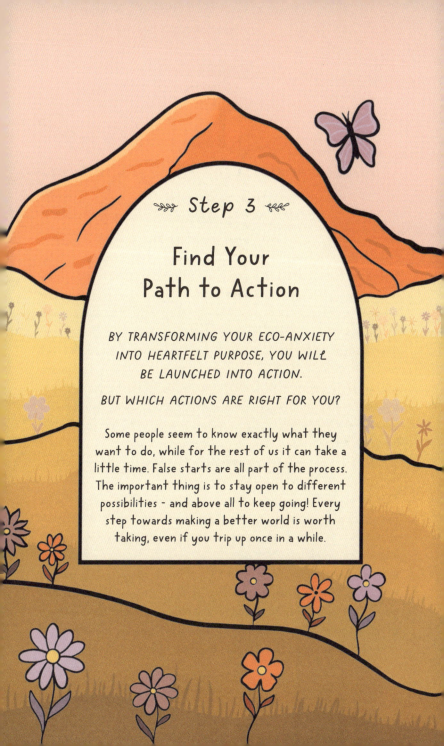

Step 3

Find Your Path to Action

BY TRANSFORMING YOUR ECO-ANXIETY INTO HEARTFELT PURPOSE, YOU WILL BE LAUNCHED INTO ACTION.

BUT WHICH ACTIONS ARE RIGHT FOR YOU?

Some people seem to know exactly what they want to do, while for the rest of us it can take a little time. False starts are all part of the process. The important thing is to stay open to different possibilities - and above all to keep going! Every step towards making a better world is worth taking, even if you trip up once in a while.

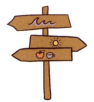

Your eco-anxiety can help you to find your purpose.

We've already said a bit about treating your eco-anxiety as a friend, but it's time to delve a little deeper. Not only can it be a friend, but also a life coach and trusted advisor. Your eco-anxiety is prodding you to take climate action. The reason it feels nasty is because it means business. It won't stop until it feels listened to. This is the science of eco-anxiety. You perceive a threat and your body wants to save you from that threat so it does all sorts of things that it thinks will help. It's hard to ignore eco-anxiety because it feels so unpleasant: that's part of its genius. It releases stress hormones into your system, which cause your heart to speed up, your blood pressure to increase, your lungs to absorb more oxygen, your pupils to widen, all of which causes your brain to think faster and your muscles to tighten.

This whole bodily chain reaction is triggered by the 'sympathetic nervous system'. When you're feeling panicky, that might not sound like the most appropriate name for it. But if you take a minute to think about it, your body is really trying to help you. In prehistoric times, that might have involved propelling you to run away from a bear. These days it may also involve propelling you to ask your parents to do the washing at a lower temperature of 20 degrees. The one thing it won't let you do is nothing. If it sees you doing nothing it will bug you until you do something.

You may be asking, but what exactly is the right thing to do? Before we answer that question, we might need to know about the parasympathetic nervous system. This is our body's natural antidote to the stress reactions we've just described. For example, once it's been established that you've successfully run away from a bear, your body sends out a new load of signals telling your heart to slow down and your breathing to return to normal. Of course this doesn't mean that your body will only give you a break once the climate crisis is fixed. Our bodies are a bit more practical than that. It's exhausting to stay in emergency mode all the time, so if your body gets the message that something is being done it will gladly take the hint. You can even slow down your breathing on purpose to tell the system to kick in. **Aren't our bodies are amazing!**

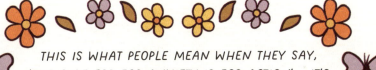

THIS IS WHAT PEOPLE MEAN WHEN THEY SAY, 'THE CURE FOR ECO-ANXIETY IS ECO-ACTION' – IT'S ACTUALLY A BIOLOGICALLY SOUND THEORY.

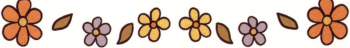

The good news is that climate action takes many, many forms. 'Action' covers everything from short-term to long-term, small acts to big acts. Anything from not eating meat on a Monday to going plastic-free, to committing to making your global corporation carbon-neutral counts. Sometimes people say, "But I can't do everything!" This is true. The point is to find a realistic position on the scale between doing nothing and doing everything.

In a sense, the first and most important thing you need to do is to acknowledge that there is a real problem. This is horrible, but it's also a genuine act of bravery. If you're reading this book, it's probably because you've already done the hard part. Go you! Once your brain and body are in agreement that something needs to be done, it becomes easier and easier to do it. . . and harder and harder not to do it!

I'm guessing you've already done this part too, but for a lot of people the next step is to look for ideas for things you can do. Eating less meat is a great idea, as people who eat a vegetarian diet tend to have a far lower carbon footprint than those of meat- or fish-eaters. Rewilding your garden is also a brilliant idea (or someone else's providing they give their permission, of course!), as you could reintroduce animals or plants that might have lived in the garden previously but do not any more. There are hundreds, if not thousands, of these things out there – so I'm not going to fill up the rest of this book by writing a list! Any or all of them are worth doing, you can just look them up and take your pick. Just remember: all climate action is worthwhile.

Lastly, when people treat environmentalists like nagging fusspots it's because they haven't understood the situation. Once you've seen the scale of the problem it stops being a pain to make small sacrifices, or to do things that require a little bravery. If there are things you can do, go for it! As you get older there will be more and more things you can do. And make sure you bring others on the journey with you – I'm sure you could teach us adults a great deal!

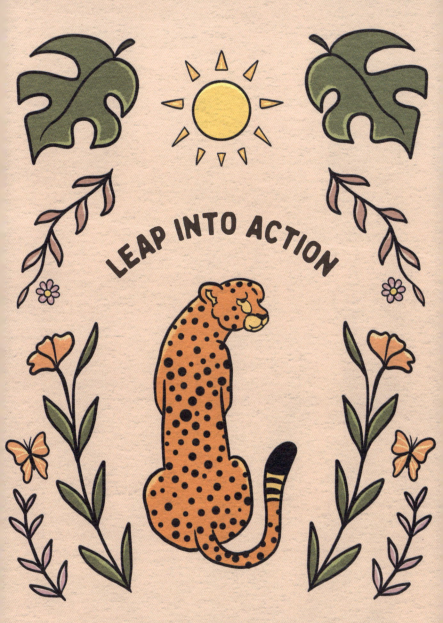

LEAP INTO ACTION

YOU'RE SO MUCH FIERCER
THAN YOU THINK

How to transform your eco-anxiety into action

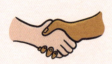

THINK OF ECO-ANXIETY AS A FRIEND

Your eco-anxiety is trying to make the world a safer place for you to live in. I like to think of it like my friend: a friend who can be annoying but you trust that they mean well.

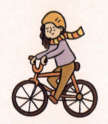

REALISE YOU DON'T HAVE TO FIX THE PROBLEM ALL AT ONCE

Start by making little changes in your personal life. And don't let people tell you there's no point. The more of us who make small differences, the more it will make a big difference.

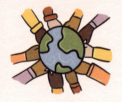

REMEMBER THAT THERE ARE A LOT OF PEOPLE LIKE YOU OUT THERE

A study from 2021 found that 75 per cent of young people said the future of the planet felt frightening. It's a clear sign that we are becoming a majority and there's real power to be found in the collective.

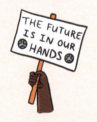

DO THE THINGS YOU CAN AND WORRY LESS ABOUT THE THINGS YOU CAN'T

It's possible to take the emergency seriously and still love life. Some people say they feel bad if they stop feeling bad. I know what they mean, but please try not to let that be you! Talking to other like-minded people, or even joining a march, can help.

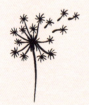

TAKE A FEW DEEP BREATHS

Even if your parasympathetic nervous system is slow to get the message, you can tell yourself that there are few actions less harmful to the planet than simply breathing.

How to find your path

FIND YOUR PEOPLE

'Activism' doesn't always have to involve a protest. There may be groups that get together just to talk and support each other, to take care of community gardens, or to go on nature-appreciating walks. You can try a few different activities and see what suits you.

INVOLVE OTHER PEOPLE

Perhaps you could get your school to celebrate Earth Day, or convince your family to do Second Hand September. Perhaps you and your friends could do a sponsored walk for charity. All of these things can be great fun and are brilliant for raising awareness.

EDUCATE YOURSELF

Food is a good place to start. Did you know that not all environmentally-aware people are vegan? There are plenty of good arguments for responsible flexitarianism. It's important to buy food that's in season and produced nearby, not flown in from hundreds of miles away.

JOIN A CLUB

Joining a club can not only help to make you feel part of a community, but these clubs are constantly coming up with new and exciting ideas for things that young people can do to combat climate change.

MAKE LONG-TERM ECO-PLANS

Maybe you will be a green town-planner or architect. I hope at least one of you will become a world leader. If people tell you there's no point in giving up eating fish, you can tell them it's just an interim plan while you work on preventing people from overfishing!

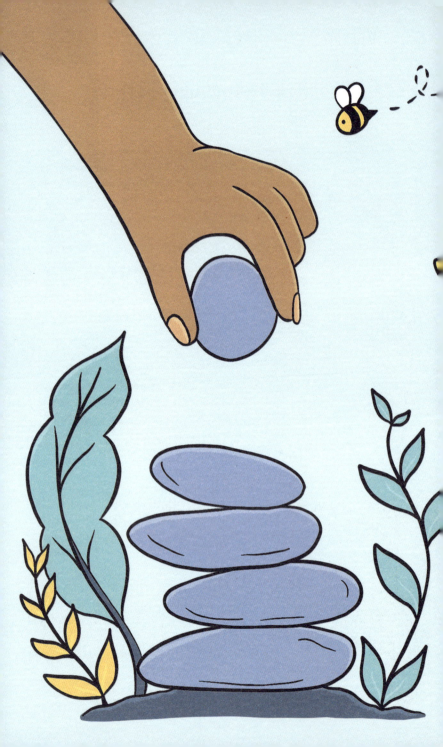

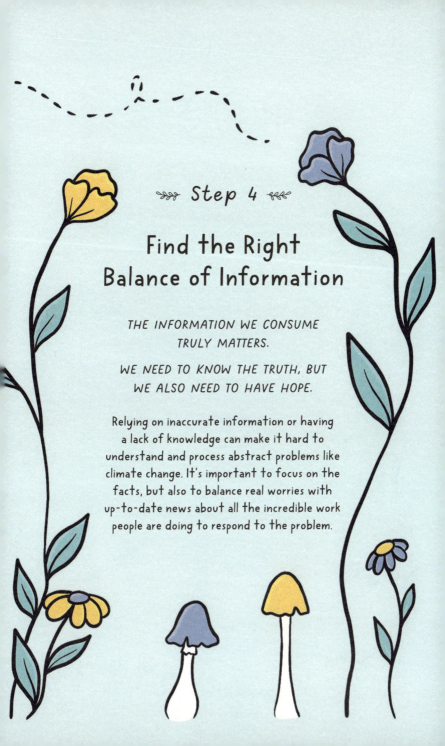

~~~ Step 4 ~~~

Find the Right Balance of Information

THE INFORMATION WE CONSUME TRULY MATTERS.

WE NEED TO KNOW THE TRUTH, BUT WE ALSO NEED TO HAVE HOPE.

Relying on inaccurate information or having a lack of knowledge can make it hard to understand and process abstract problems like climate change. It's important to focus on the facts, but also to balance real worries with up-to-date news about all the incredible work people are doing to respond to the problem.

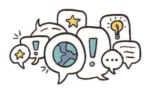

How do we know what's true?

It's all very well to say, 'follow the science' and, 'listen to the facts' but how do we know who's telling the truth? For a start, not all scientists agree with each other. Different scientists might care about one aspect of climate change more than another and as a result they might disagree about which theory is better. After all, there are many types of climate scientists working across different fields - such as meteorology (study of the earth's atmosphere and weather), biochemistry (the chemistry of living organisms) and geophysics (the earth's physical processes) - and scientists in different fields have different ideas about how we should be responding to climate change. Should we focus on global food systems, fuel use or manufacturing? Or is it only any use if we think of all three at once? It's all very well to believe our current political and economic systems are no longer fit for purpose and say, 'We want system change, not climate change,' but scientists don't all agree on which new systems would be most effective.

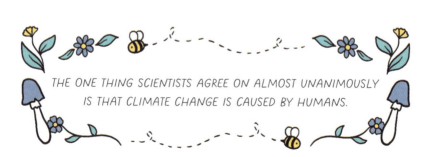

THE ONE THING SCIENTISTS AGREE ON ALMOST UNANIMOUSLY IS THAT CLIMATE CHANGE IS CAUSED BY HUMANS.

In 2021, research involving 90,000 climate-related studies found that 99.9 per cent of scientists agreed that anthropogenic (human-related) climate change is real. The lead author on the study came out and said, "It is really case closed. There is nobody of significance in the scientific community who doubts human-caused climate change." The reason they used the phrase 'case closed' is because the rapid rise of social media in the last decade brought with it a surge in climate misinformation from people whose business it was to make science look like opinion. These people are known as climate-change deniers. Thankfully, as time goes on, climate-change deniers are being caught out and it's becoming more and more difficult to spread lies about climate change. Some mainstream news outlets may be frustratingly uninterested when it comes to climate change, but at least the stories that appear there should be properly fact-checked. Social media, however, isn't regulated in this way and is still pretty much the Wild West where climate information is concerned.

If you've picked up this book, I know you'll agree it's important to listen to the scientists, not people on social media. But I want to tell you that it's fine to not listen to them all the time! Sometimes we might rather listen to music, or the birdsong outside. The newspaper I read, for example, aims to report consistently and responsibly about climate change. This means there are numerous upsetting articles every day that sometimes make me feel sick with worry. I regularly skip that section if I'm not in the mood to digest it there and then. **Remember, if there's an important new piece of information, it will always reach you somehow - it won't just disappear from the news after one day.**

Once you're engaged with the climate crisis, you don't need to absorb every new bit of proof that the world is at risk. This is not going to make you a better environmentalist, it's just going to make you very unhappy. So be kind to yourself and tell yourself it's OK to switch off the news and open your eyes and ears to other things. It's all about balance.

Plus, on the bright side, people all over the world are working really hard to slow down climate change. There are scientists, activists, politicians, Indigenous Elders, business people, young people, plants, insects, all doing everything in their power to sustain a healthy planet. We need to hear their stories too. Cristiana Figueres, who was instrumental in bringing about the Paris Climate Agreement (which aims to keep the world below 1.5 degrees of warming), has coined the term 'stubborn optimism' to describe a constructive attitude towards the future of the environment. **We mustn't give in to pessimism as this might stop us fighting to make important changes.** But you have to be stubborn to be an optimist when there's so much bad news around!

Not only will good news make you feel better, it will help you to cultivate the kind of mental attitude most likely to make a positive difference to the world. One easy way to get a dose of optimism is simply to tap the words 'good climate news' into a search engine. I just did this and learned that in the future aeroplanes might be designed to run on sugar-eating bacteria, that surgeons are developing climate-friendly operations and that dolphin poo may hold the key to saving coral reefs!

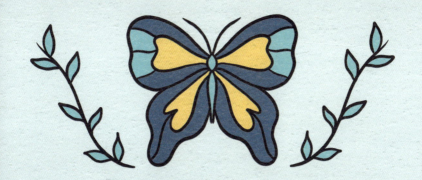

REMEMBER THAT
READING GOOD NEWS IS
JUST AS IMPORTANT AS
READING BAD NEWS

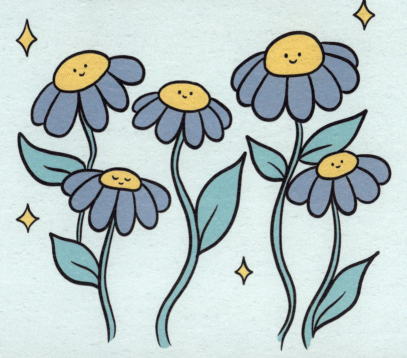

Climate change resources

WWW.CLIMATEKIDS.NASA.GOV

NASA Climate Kids is the United States space agency's website explaining climate change and provides simple explanations of complex problems. If you feel like you're only just beginning to see the links between cars and polar bears, or avocados and rivers, then this is a great place to start.

WWW.DOGONEWS.COM

Dogo News is a bilingual kids' news website that you can read in English or Spanish. It has an environment section, as well as science, social studies, world news and what they call 'civics', which means stories about people. The great thing about this website is that it's uncompromising and not at all patronising.

WWW.KIDS.NATIONALGEOGRAPHIC.COM

National Geographic Kids is a magazine with a focus on the natural world. They also have a fantastic website, with different pages featuring different parts of the world.

WWW.KIDSNEWS.COM.AU

Kids News is a Australian news website where you can choose the complexity of articles to match your reading age. It's important to listen to what the Australians have to say about the environment as, like many countries, it is on the front line of climate change.

WWW.TIMEFORKIDS.COM

Time Magazine devotes a section of their website to news tailored especially to children. They cover all sorts of news, not just environmental, so you can also read international science, history and community news stories.

How to fuel your 'stubborn optimism'

TRUST THE 99.9 PER CENT OF SCIENTISTS

Not only are they in agreement about the reality of the climate emergency, but many of them are busy working on solutions. It's normal that they should have different ideas from one another - the more ideas the better!

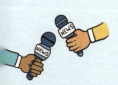

STAY INFORMED

Rather than being drowned by the daily drip of bad news, just stay informed about the big picture. Every six to seven years, the Intergovernmental Panel on Climate Change (IPCC) issues a report on climate change and you can read simple summaries online.

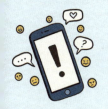

ALLOW YOURSELF TO SWITCH OFF

Some people act like listening to the news every day is compulsory, but it isn't. It can be healthy to do other stuff instead. A study from 2013 found that watching the news can decrease your creativity - and what this planet needs is creative people, so learn to switch it off!

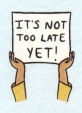

REJECT THE TERM 'DOOMER'

This is an unhelpful word that can be used to shut down anyone who's concerned about the impact of climate change. If anyone calls you a doomer, refer them to the latest IPCC report. Do they think they know better than the many thousands of specialists who produced it?

SEEK OUT POSITIVE STORIES

Instead of sitting passively in front of the evening news, take control of the information you consume and search for something nice for a change! This is not running away, this is fuelling your determination for tomorrow.

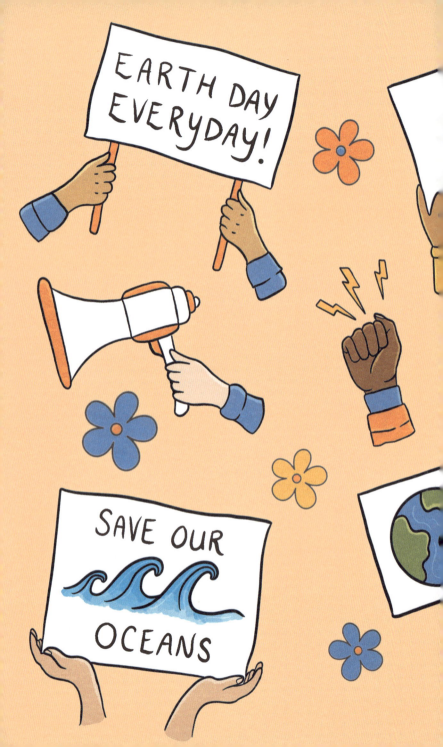

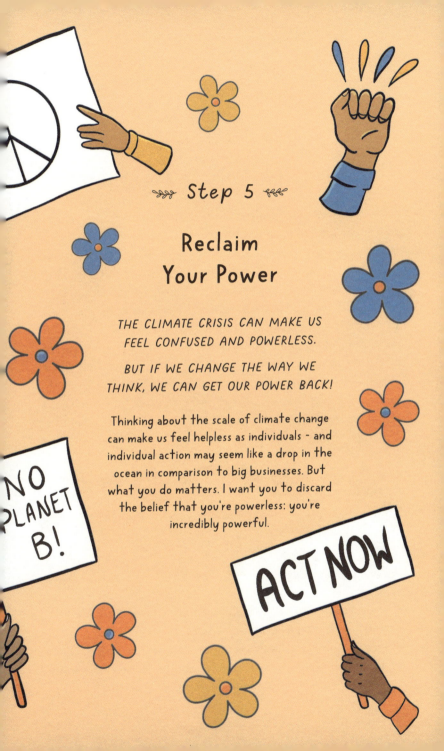

≫≫≫ Step 5 *≪≪≪*

Reclaim
Your Power

*THE CLIMATE CRISIS CAN MAKE US
FEEL CONFUSED AND POWERLESS.*

*BUT IF WE CHANGE THE WAY WE
THINK, WE CAN GET OUR POWER BACK!*

Thinking about the scale of climate change
can make us feel helpless as individuals - and
individual action may seem like a drop in the
ocean in comparison to big businesses. But
what you do matters. I want you to discard
the belief that you're powerless: you're
incredibly powerful.

NO
PLANET
B!

ACT NOW

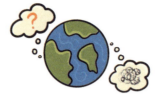

It's time to clear up climate confusion.

Putting the climate deniers aside, even environmentalists can give mixed messaging about what we should be doing to avert the climate crisis. Some people say the best thing we can do is to stop flying, others say to switch to a plant-based diet. But then again you will hear some people say that individual action is pointless if massive change doesn't happen at a societal level. So, who's right? Maybe it's helpful to understand a little bit more about why some environmentalists are less keen on the idea of individual action. It's certainly not because they think eating less meat and using less fossil fuel are bad ideas. They are just questioning the notion that each of us should be taking full responsibility for the climate in our private lives while some governments and big businesses don't play their part.

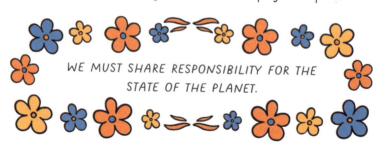

WE MUST SHARE RESPONSIBILITY FOR THE STATE OF THE PLANET.

If we all feel like we're privately responsible, then it can make the problem seem insoluble, which leads to despair and guilt, because we can never do enough. This not only makes us feel awful, it allows those big organisations to carry on making money while polluting our world. How unfair is that?

Instead of trying to solve the problem of whether we should be cutting out meat or cancelling our summer holiday abroad, we would be better off saying we can do either or both. It's all worthwhile. This doesn't mean we have to be performing all manner of environmental action at all times! This is another one of those unhelpful thought patterns that just makes us feel bad. It's much more productive to think that we'll do what we can when we can. And, if we act together, we can do a lot.

While environmentalists who say we ought to be focusing all our energy on massive societal change surely mean well, their message risks playing into the hands of the very people they are hoping to challenge. If we all stopped recycling and started eating beef for every meal, would that give us any more time or resources to lobby for change? No! But would it give governments and big businesses an excuse to say, "Why should we care about the planet when no one else seems to?" Yes, it would!

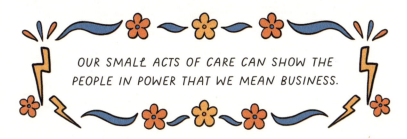

OUR SMALL ACTS OF CARE CAN SHOW THE PEOPLE IN POWER THAT WE MEAN BUSINESS.

There are many more of us than there are of them. **If we all act according to our principles it forces the powerful people to listen to us.** If our governments do things we disapprove of, we won't vote for them. If businesses do things we disappove of, we won't buy their products. So, who's got the power now?

The idea that we have to choose between the personal and the political is wrong. I think it's much more sensible to follow the feminists of the 1960s who said, "The personal is political." What we do in our private lives matters on the grand scale: there's a real strength in numbers. If we all agree we'd like a habitable planet, then we can bring about monumental change by living in sustainable ways, and creating virtuous circles where our own actions lend support and impetus to the actions of others. Social scientists agree that our individual actions on climate have significant effects on the behaviour of the people around us.

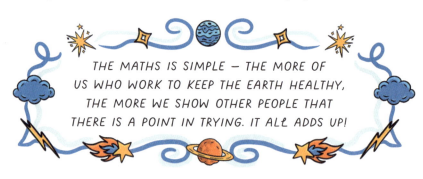

THE MATHS IS SIMPLE — THE MORE OF US WHO WORK TO KEEP THE EARTH HEALTHY, THE MORE WE SHOW OTHER PEOPLE THAT THERE IS A POINT IN TRYING. IT ALL ADDS UP!

We hear a lot about negative tipping points - moments beyond which icebergs can't stay frozen, or insect species can't reproduce. But we need to start working towards positive tipping points, where entire populations stop buying from polluting businesses and withdraw support from leaders who fail to protect our precious ecosystems. If we keep pushing in the right direction, we can make ourselves part of a powerful mass. Huge numbers of people doing small things can be more powerful than a few people doing big things. And all sorts of people doing all manner of environmentally responsible things, big and small, is the very best option of all.

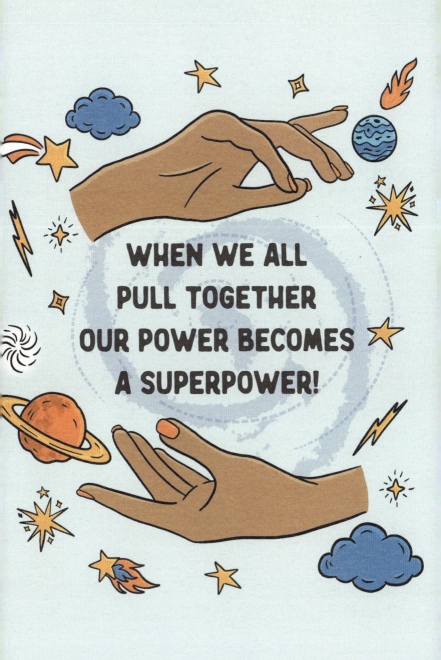

WHEN WE ALL
PULL TOGETHER
OUR POWER BECOMES
A SUPERPOWER!

Eco-friendly activities

Given that none of us is likely to become prime minister anytime soon, we have to learn to make the best use of the powers we have. Get a notepad and pen and make a list of some things you can do to help slow down climate change.

HERE ARE SOME IDEAS:

 Walk rather than taking the car whenever possible

 Plant wildflowers to help butterflies and bees

 Avoid single-use, disposable items

 Switch off appliances when you're not using them

 Save energy and water by being quick in the shower

That's a great start already. Now, take your list and see how you could turbo-charge it. First of all, ask yourself which groups or organisations you are a part of. This can be anything from your family to your football team. Are there ways you can involve other people in fighting climate change?

 Could you get everyone on your street to turn off their home electronic devices when they aren't using them?

 Could you take control of the school garden to make it a refuge for insects?

 Could you get your football team to use re-usable water bottles?

How to cultivate your power

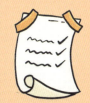

RAISE AWARENESS

If you make a list of actions and bring other people on board, not only will there be more people doing those actions, you will be showing them how it's possible to make a difference. With luck, they'll soon be making lists of their own.

TRY TO MAKE IT FUN

One myth about environmentalists is that we're gloomy people who want to spoil everyone else's fun, when actually we love the planet and want to preserve the possibility of fun for eternity! When you're trying to involve other people, do whatever you can to make sure they have a good time.

BE AMBITIOUS

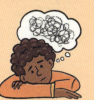

Treat getting people on board like a video game with ascending levels. For example, if you get your parents to agree to switch to an ethical bank account - one which aims to have no negative impact on the environment - maybe you could then suggest that the companies they work for do the same.

DON'T BE PUT OFF BY FAILURE

It's not always easy to do this stuff. Sometimes you have to have ten ideas in order to make just one of them a reality. Having positive hopes can fuel your motivation to persevere.

WHEN YOU FIND YOUR POWER, (OAT) MILK IT!

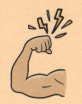

Perhaps your special power will be to make delicious plant-based meals that convert all your friends. Or maybe you will use your child-charm to make older people listen. Child-charm is the not-so-secret weapon of the environmental movement. Use it before you grow up!

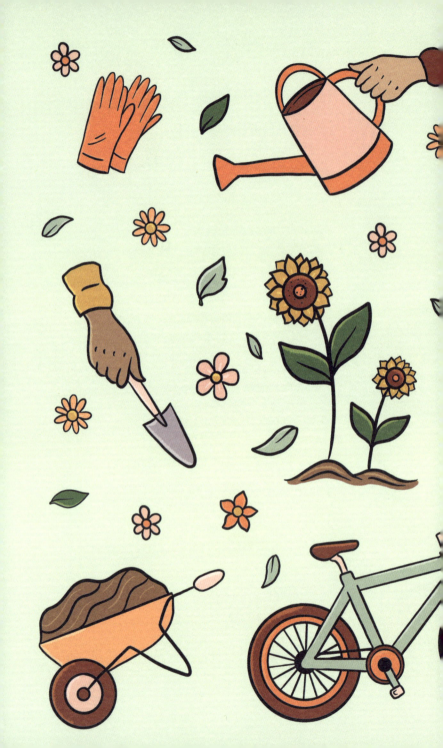

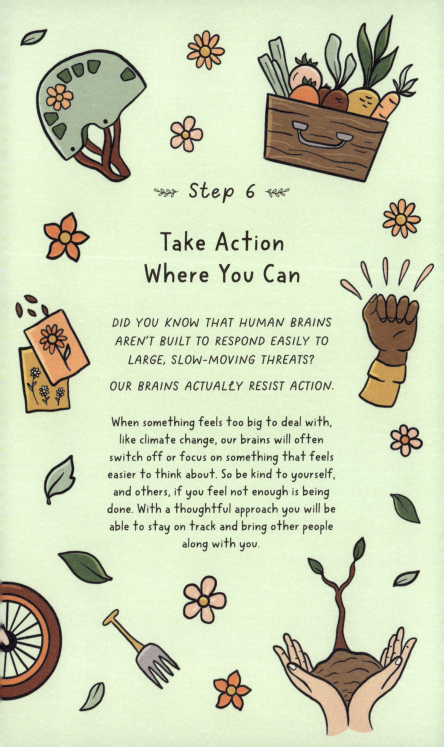

Step 6

Take Action
Where You Can

DID YOU KNOW THAT HUMAN BRAINS AREN'T BUILT TO RESPOND EASILY TO LARGE, SLOW-MOVING THREATS?

OUR BRAINS ACTUALLY RESIST ACTION.

When something feels too big to deal with, like climate change, our brains will often switch off or focus on something that feels easier to think about. So be kind to yourself, and others, if you feel not enough is being done. With a thoughtful approach you will be able to stay on track and bring other people along with you.

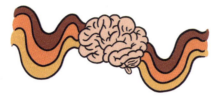

Not all minds think alike.

Most human brains are brilliant at reacting to fast-moving threats. For example, if a ball is flying straight towards your head, you might find yourself jumping out of the way before you've had even a second to think about it. Slow threats, however, are much better at getting around our built-in alarm systems. This is because we're always processing such huge amounts of information that we tend to focus on the things that require our immediate attention. However, some of us seem to be more inclined to react to slow threats than others. **People with eco-anxiety are more willing and more able to consider distant hazards.**

The human brain generally is much more able to deal with certainty than uncertainty because responding to uncertainty often requires more complex calculations. Although we are now certain that climate change is real, we can't predict exactly how and when it will unfold. The human brain is constantly weeding out information in order to avoid brain-overload. If it tried to plan for absolutely everything it would soon go into meltdown! **However people with eco-anxiety are more ready to allow for uncertainty without trying to shut it down.** The downside of this is that, having understood the scale of the climate emergency, it can become **ALL** we can think about. It's as if the only possible reactions are indifference or panic, and this isn't good for our mind or body. Luckily for our mental health, this isn't the case. We can focus on some more positive features of our incredible human brains. Not only can they react very fast in order to save us from immediate threats, but they are also good at working out difficult problems and imagining various futures.

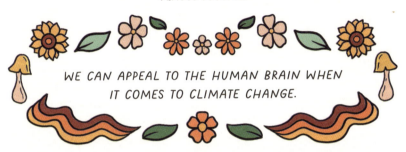

WE CAN APPEAL TO THE HUMAN BRAIN WHEN IT COMES TO CLIMATE CHANGE.

We are able to understand why it's happening and we are also perfectly capable of understanding what we need to do to stop it. For example, we know we need to give up over-consuming harmful oil and gas and switch to cleaner, renewable energy sources. And we know this because the brains of brilliant scientists have consistently come to this conclusion.

Of course that makes it sound a bit too easy! In order to do that millions of people would have to get on board. The good news is that even the most resistant people finally seem to be grasping the idea that something needs to be done. If the climate crisis is like a ball travelling towards our heads in extreme slow motion, it's close enough now that even the slow-reactors are realising it's going to hurt if we don't do something and fast. Perhaps we could say that this historical moment has something in common with a forest fire. It will just take a few bright sparks to ignite humanity's passion to get on with the job. And maybe one of those sparks is you!

If the best hope we have of making a difference is to galvanise as many people as possible into action, then we must be clever about how we present the problem. Even if our unhelpful inner critic is telling us, "It's a total disaster! Everyone's useless! It's too late!" we have to tell it to give us a minute while we think of a more inspiring message.

The good thing about the human brain is that it's always trying to work out what's best for us. Sometimes it miscalculates and chooses things that are good in the short-term but bad in the long-term - like eating sweets instead of vegetables! If you tell people that the world will soon be destroyed, they might very well decide to have a party on the way out. But if you explain to them that we can actually make a big difference in a short time then they will be far more likely to respond constructively. The vast majority of people really do agree that the best thing for all of us is to take care of the only world we've got. It's pretty much a no-brainer.

I'd like you to visualise yourself as a tiny spark of pure energy. Tell yourself you're going to use this energy to fire up everyone you meet. When people see the passion you put into making a better world, they'll join forces and together you'll burn even brighter. We know how to save our wonderful planet - so let's get on with it!

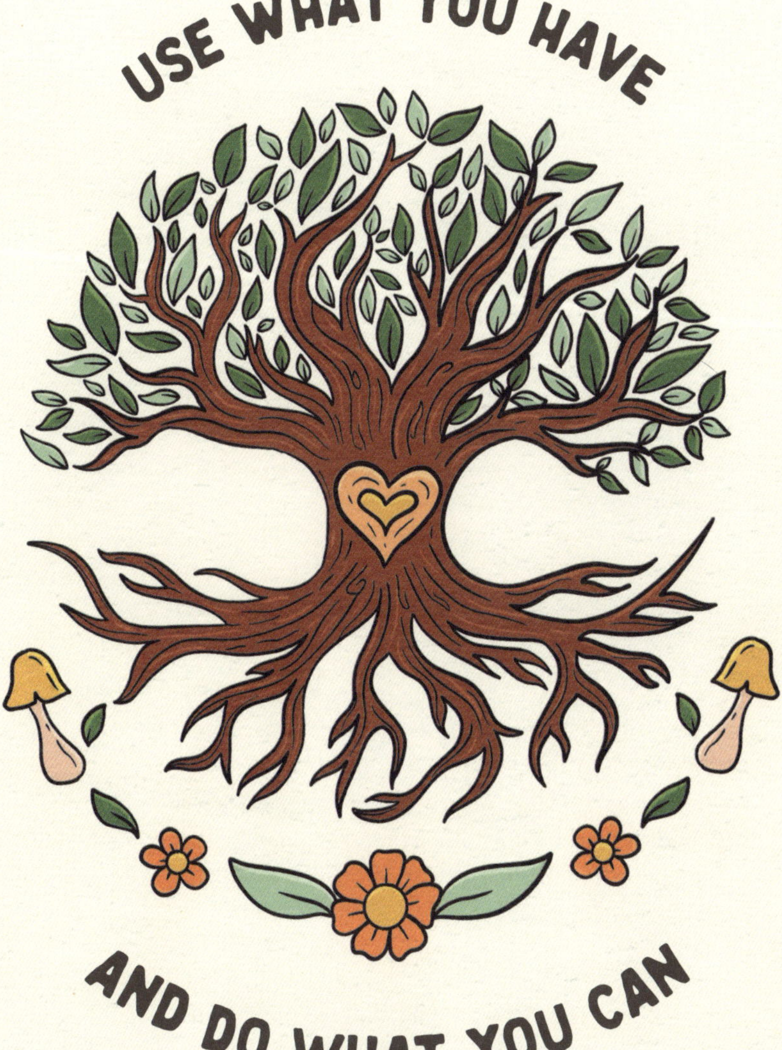

Learn something new

Give your brilliant brain a treat. These five documentaries are packed full of extraordinary ideas, knowledge and inspiration to help you turn your thoughts into actions:

1 2040

A positive documentary about what we could achieve using existing ideas and technology to counteract climate change. Made by a father who gives us a hopeful vision of what it's possible to achieve by the time his children grow up.

2 BEFORE THE FLOOD

Film star Leonardo di Caprio takes us on a journey to learn about the climate emergency. We meet scientists who teach us the science behind climate change and we also learn about the possible solutions.

3 I AM GRETA

A close-up portrait of the globally famous teenage climate activist, Greta Thunberg. This one's great as it shows Greta as both a regular young person and as someone who can stand up to some of the most powerful adults in the world.

4 LIVING ON ONE DOLLAR

A group of friends go to rural Guatemala to find out what it's like to live on a dollar a day, as 1.1 billion people on the planet currently do. Rather than simply showing how these people might need our help, it also shows how we need theirs.

5 OUR PLANET

Narrated by David Attenborough, this eight-part series looks at the ways in which human activities are affecting wildlife all over the world. You could watch an episode a week in a climate action group, or alternate episodes with activities every other week.

Set up a climate action group

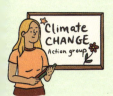

GET AT LEAST ONE TEACHER ON SIDE

They will be able to help you with practicalities - like when and where to have meetings. You will also need the school's permission to set up the group.

SPREAD THE WORD

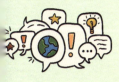

Stick up flyers or put a notice in the school newsletter to let everyone know you're setting up a climate action group. Give plenty of notice so that everyone who wants to be there can make it. Decide whether you'd like to include parents or just kids. Maybe you could even have your own parents' evenings!

MAKE A PLAN FOR YOUR FIRST MEETING

It's very important that the people who turn up feel that there is a point in being there. Action is the key word here! Suggest some activities that you could all do together - write letters, invite speakers, raise money, put on an assembly, organise petitions, make banners, join protests, watch films, make films, produce your own newsletter and so on.

KEEP MOMENTUM GOING

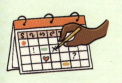

End each meeting with a really good plan for the next one. Some groups fizzle out if it feels like no one knows what they're doing. Always aim to give people a reason to come back. Having lots of well-structured activities will make it fun as well as purposeful.

USE SOCIAL MEDIA

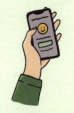

With the help of an adult, make a YouTube video, or even a TikTok. Anything to get your message out there. Who knows, you might even end up as a positive climate story on the evening news!

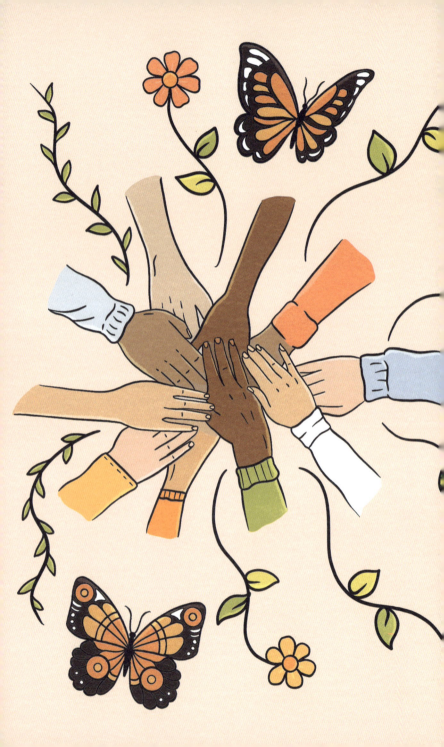

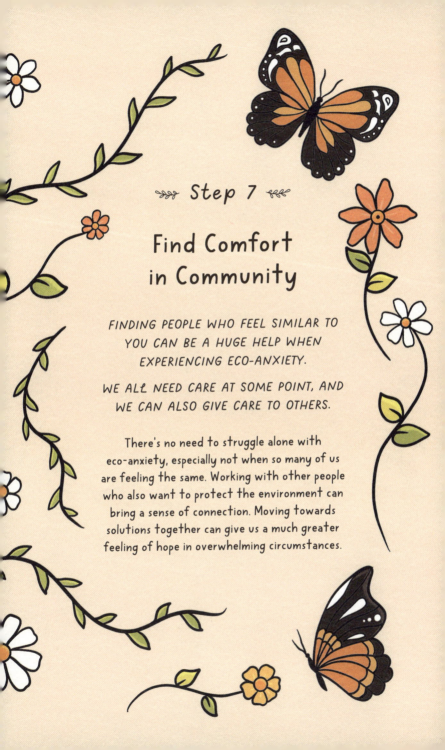

*** Step 7 ***

Find Comfort in Community

FINDING PEOPLE WHO FEEL SIMILAR TO YOU CAN BE A HUGE HELP WHEN EXPERIENCING ECO-ANXIETY.

WE ALL NEED CARE AT SOME POINT, AND WE CAN ALSO GIVE CARE TO OTHERS.

There's no need to struggle alone with eco-anxiety, especially not when so many of us are feeling the same. Working with other people who also want to protect the environment can bring a sense of connection. Moving towards solutions together can give us a much greater feeling of hope in overwhelming circumstances.

A safe space is a place where you feel safe to be honest.

I've shared a lot in this book about staying optimistic and sending out positive messages, but what about the times when we feel really sad, angry and hopeless? These are real feelings, with real causes, so they need a real outlet. It's no good keeping our faces frozen into smiles while we're feeling horrible inside.

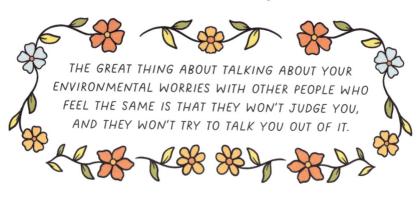

THE GREAT THING ABOUT TALKING ABOUT YOUR ENVIRONMENTAL WORRIES WITH OTHER PEOPLE WHO FEEL THE SAME IS THAT THEY WON'T JUDGE YOU, AND THEY WON'T TRY TO TALK YOU OUT OF IT.

There is an eco-philosopher called Timothy Morton who coined the phrase 'the ecological thought'. It means the moment when you realise that all is not well with the environment on a truly momentous, complex scale. 'Thought' doesn't even quite feel like the right word for it - it's just so huge. Once you've had this thought it would be very, very difficult to unthink it. You can't go backwards, so you just have to keep going forwards.

People who have had 'the ecological thought' are well-equipped to be kind to one another. We all know what it's like to feel the panic and grief that comes with understanding the damage that's being done to our world. If we know that someone else is feeling this way too our hearts immediately go out to them.

There are so many reasons to open up and share feelings. If people don't know how you feel, they won't be able to help you, which is not only bad for you, it's bad for them, too. It's terrible when you can see that someone feels sad but you have no idea why. If people know you're having a hard time they can validate your feelings and they might also help you to see things slightly differently. There's also the unfortunate fact that bad feelings have a habit of hanging around until you acknowledge them. Ignoring them doesn't necessarily make them go away. You'll be amazed to see how helpful it is to share your feelings with someone else who's had 'the ecological thought'.

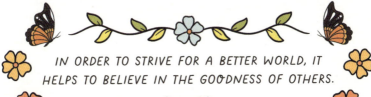

IN ORDER TO STRIVE FOR A BETTER WORLD, IT HELPS TO BELIEVE IN THE GOODNESS OF OTHERS.

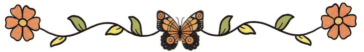

When you share your difficult feelings with other people you are giving them a chance to take care of you. You don't need to feel that you are asking a favour or adding a burden. Not only will you feel less alone, but so will the people you're sharing with. It's lovely to be there for one another and one day you will be able to take care of someone else who's suffering.

Building communities of like-minded people is helpful for increasing momentum and showing it's possible to act positively. But what about the people who don't seem so bothered? It can be easy to get cross with them and to blame them for all the world's problems, but it isn't really their fault. Also, if we want them to join us in our fight against climate change it's important that we don't start too many arguments with them!

We need to find a balance between seeking out people we can share our feelings with honestly and keeping a place open for people who don't feel the same way, or who are just a few steps behind. 'The ecological thought' is very uncomfortable in the beginning, and perhaps not everyone is ready to have it. But once you've had it you can start to learn to live with it, and even to find a certain peace in the idea that at least now you know you can do something about it.

By being there with and for other people who are ready and willing to take care of the planet, we can demonstrate to everyone that it's OK to acknowledge the uncomfortable truth. We have to go through a painful period of mental adjustment, but in the end it's better than trying to pretend it isn't happening. It's always inspiring to meet other people who have let themselves confront the agonising realities of climate change but are still capable of happiness, kindness and optimism.

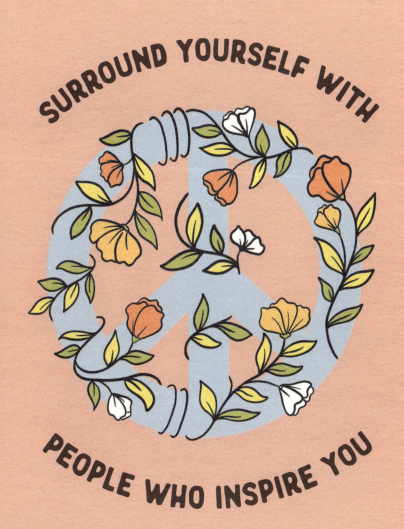

SURROUND YOURSELF WITH

PEOPLE WHO INSPIRE YOU

Climate Café

Have you heard of Climate Cafés? They happen all around the world and they show people they are not alone in their fears.

WHAT IS A CLIMATE CAFÉ?

A Climate Café is a place where anyone can come to discuss thoughts and feelings about the climate emergency. The focus is on conversation rather than actions or solutions, which makes it different from a climate action group.

CAN ANYONE GO?

Many Climate Cafés are for over-18s, so you'd need to look for one that welcomes younger people. Other than that, they aim to be as inclusive as possible.

WHERE CAN I FIND ONE?

You could look online for 'Climate Cafés near me' or go to **www.climateandmind.org**. Alternatively, you could ask an adult to help you set one up for the people in your community. You can find brilliant tips on hosting Climate Cafés online at **www.climatecafés.org/home/hosting-climate-cafés**.

WHAT'S THE POINT IN JUST TALKING?

The idea behind Climate Cafés is that, as we see the effects of climate change, more and more people will need to process their feelings around it. If we sense we are alone with these difficult feelings, not only will we suffer them more, but we will feel powerless to act. But after having had a good chat, we might then feel empowered to go and do something about it!

WHAT IF I'M TOO SHY?

It can be hard to talk about upsetting ideas in front of a group of people. The whole point in Climate Cafés is to be as welcoming and accepting as possible. It's a safe space and people find them inspiring, positive places to go along to.

How to be a good listener

When we feel upset, we often turn to others for help and support. So when others come to us in pain, we should do our best to help them feel better by listening to them.

1 GIVE THE OTHER PERSON TIME

Sometimes it's difficult to find the right words for things. It can even take a few tries. Be patient if the person who's speaking doesn't get to the point straight away.

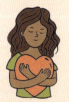

2 SHOW INTEREST

There's nothing worse than speaking to someone who looks bored or like they'd rather be doing something else. You can show interest through your body language, like looking the person who's speaking in the eye.

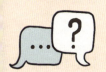

3 ASK QUESTIONS

This is not only a great way to express interest, but it can help the other person to think in new ways. We can sometimes surprise ourselves with what we learn, too!

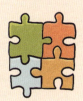

4 DON'T TRY TO SOLVE EVERYTHING

When people are upset it can be tempting to rush in with solutions, but if it's obvious stuff that they've probably already thought of it won't help much and they might even get annoyed. It's enough that you're being kind and listening, you don't have to fix everything as well!

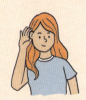

5 LISTEN WITHOUT JUDGING

Try to focus on listening, rather than reacting. If you start reacting emotionally to what's being said, then it can get in the way of listening to what is said next. Other people's unhappiness can be overwhelming, so if you're really worried about a friend, tell a responsible adult – don't feel you have to cope with it all by yourself.

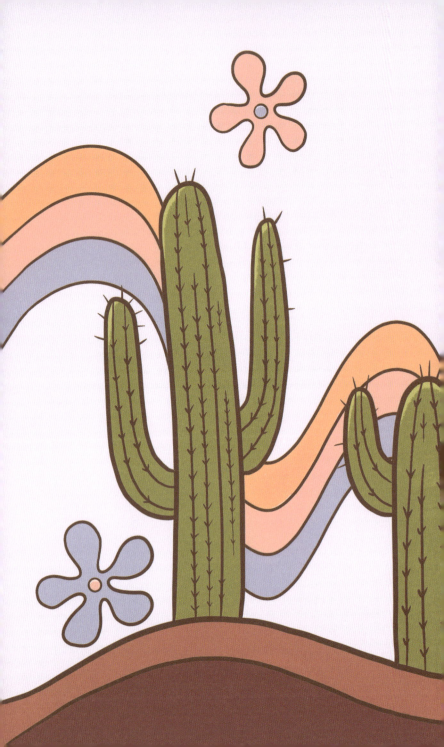

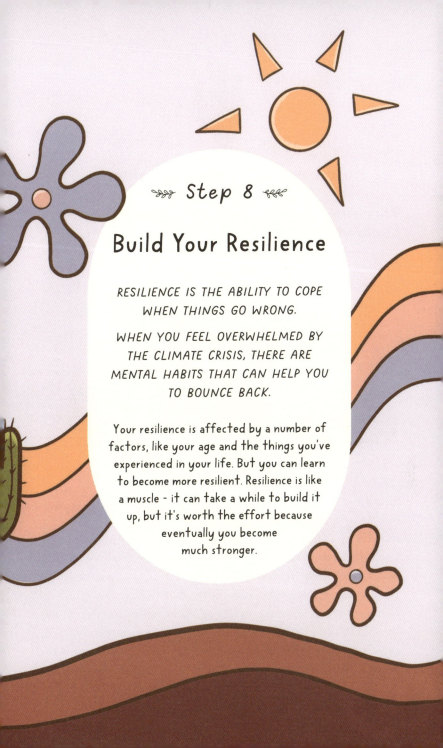

Step 8

Build Your Resilience

RESILIENCE IS THE ABILITY TO COPE WHEN THINGS GO WRONG.

WHEN YOU FEEL OVERWHELMED BY THE CLIMATE CRISIS, THERE ARE MENTAL HABITS THAT CAN HELP YOU TO BOUNCE BACK.

Your resilience is affected by a number of factors, like your age and the things you've experienced in your life. But you can learn to become more resilient. Resilience is like a muscle - it can take a while to build it up, but it's worth the effort because eventually you become much stronger.

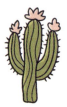

How can I build up my resilience?

We can learn resilience from wind-resistant plants. Some plants, like palms and conifers, are very good at growing in windy places. They tend to have bendy stems and narrow leaves so they can flex and sway without getting knocked over. So, just like palms and conifers, rather than staying stiff and still, we can cultivate supple ways of thinking and adapting to new situations.

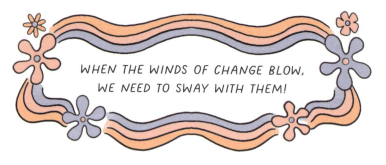

WHEN THE WINDS OF CHANGE BLOW, WE NEED TO SWAY WITH THEM!

In order to become more resilient, we have to learn to cope better with uncertainty. As we've already seen in Step 6, this is sometimes easier said than done. Still, anyone who remembers living through the COVID-19 pandemic knows that the whole world can change in the space of a few weeks, and that it's possible to find ways to move with it. Although the COVID-19 pandemic was extremely hard for many, many people, it also showed that we can find ingenious ways to survive extraordinary events. While millions of us were shut in our houses for months on end, we still often found things to do. Maybe we grew our own food or wrote letters to our friends. Perhaps some of us even came out of it a little wiser! One of the greatest forms of resilience is to be able to find happiness in unusual circumstances - and the pandemic certainly provided lots of opportunities to practice just that.

Situations like the COVID-19 pandemic teach us that the world operates independently of our wills and wishes. We might want one thing and get another. The thing about living in an industrialised society is that we are led to expect so many aspects of our lives to remain stable and under our control. Our houses keep us warm in winter and cool in summer. Fresh fruits and vegetables are available year-round. Not only that, but our economic systems are designed to give us the impression that everything is running smoothly, even when it isn't. It's hardly surprising that so many of us are so terrified of change. But this is not a healthy way to live.

Although we don't know exactly how and when climate change will begin to seriously affect us, we can be fairly sure it will. And of course if we are involved in the fight to slow it down, that would suggest we see the changes as undesirable. Still, this doesn't mean the future will be horrible. It will be different, for sure, but different isn't always bad. I'm certainly not saying, 'Climate change doesn't matter because we will adapt.' **It's more that, given we know it's happening, we need to trust we will apply our ingenuity to the new challenges we face.** In a sense, life is resilience. Plants grow, wounds heal, species adapt. Life bends to new circumstances. This is what we mean when we say, 'life force'. Life itself seems to want to keep going.

Rather than thinking we need all the same material advantages and comforts as our parents had, we have to acknowledge that this probably won't happen. And that it will be OK. All the technology, money and medicine that we take for granted is in some ways quite unusual. Not only did humans manage without them for many thousands of years, lots of people around the world still do.

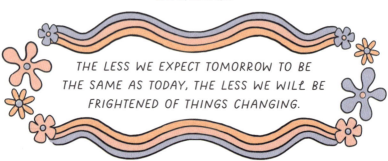

THE LESS WE EXPECT TOMORROW TO BE THE SAME AS TODAY, THE LESS WE WILL BE FRIGHTENED OF THINGS CHANGING.

Maybe they'll only change a little bit. Maybe they'll change a lot. Perhaps some things will change for the better and some for the worse. We really have no idea. For younger people living through the climate crisis, it can be hard to know how to think about the future. Not only do older people have the advantage of not having so much future ahead of them, but our life experiences often tell us that even really terrible difficulties can be overcome. Sometimes, the thing you most dread actually happens and sometimes you recover from it. But like any plant, however weather-resistant, it helps to have strong foundations, like good soil and water. So, let's use the toolkit on the next page to lay the groundwork so that we can grow into the most resilient creatures we can be...

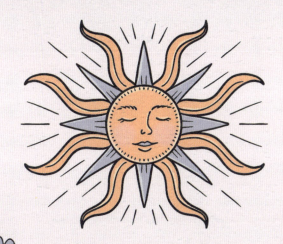

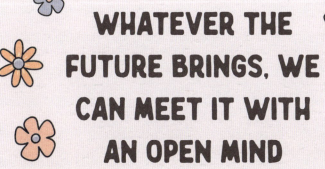

WHATEVER THE FUTURE BRINGS, WE CAN MEET IT WITH AN OPEN MIND

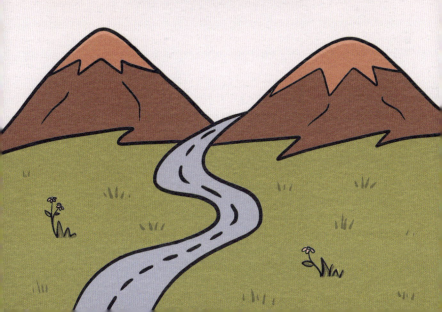

Thought patterns to let go of

Here are some unhelpful habits that work against resilience and how we can reframe them to manage our eco-anxiety.

CATASTROPHISING

This means thinking of the worst-case scenario and acting like it's definitely going to happen. Remember that not only do we not know what will happen in the future, but sometimes bad things happen and people respond brilliantly.

HOPELESSNESS

This one's terrible as it has the double-whammy effect of making us sad in the present as well as making it less likely that we will try to make things better. Hope is necessary for change - keep yours alive and invest in a brighter future.

GUILT

The climate crisis is not your fault! If we were born into an industrial society, we will have done any number of non-climate-friendly things. We're all in the process of dealing with this - it's not just on you.

RUMINATIONS

Sometimes our thoughts get stuck in a loop, like a cow endlessly digesting the same mouthfuls of grass. This tends to happen with problems we can't solve - we keep going back to them as if it will be different this time. Tell yourself that the thoughts you're having are already making a difference to how you act and that's plenty for now.

RAGE

It's easy to feel angry when you think of the people who are harming the planet for profit. But our climate actions can be powered by love instead of hate. Not only will it be better for us in the short term, but it will also allow us to welcome more people into the climate movement in the long term.

Five pillars of resilience

1 REST

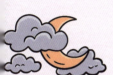

It's much harder to regulate your moods when you're tired. Resting is also one of the most eco-friendly activities in the world, so do it as much as you need to. Also, for the insomniacs among you, don't worry about lying awake once in a while as time spent resting in bed is 60 per cent as good as actual sleep.

2 HEALTH

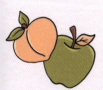

Physical health is also very important for mood-regulation and energy levels. Even simple exercise, like going for a walk, can release happiness hormones into your system. Also, eating a plant-heavy diet can be good for individual health as well as planetary health.

3 AGENCY

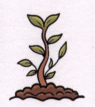

This means having the sense that the things you do can make a difference. Sometimes it takes a bit of trial and error to work out what works and what doesn't. But even if all you can do for now is to make small changes in your own life, that's wonderful. As you grow up you will begin to access more and more ways to act on the Earth's behalf.

4 COMMUNITY

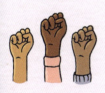

Having a network of friends and family is not only helpful for mental stability, but also for taking bigger actions and making more effective changes. However, not all of us have a massive crowd of friends, or a stable, loving family. It can take time to find your people, but never lose hope. And on that subject...

5 ACTIVE HOPE

Passive hope - crossing your fingers and hoping for the best - isn't going to solve the crisis. But active hope very well might! If we have the hope that we can make things better, then it will always seem worthwhile to keep trying.

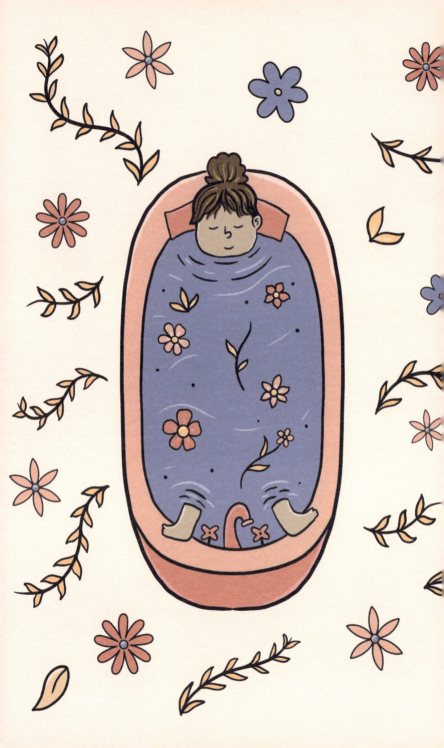

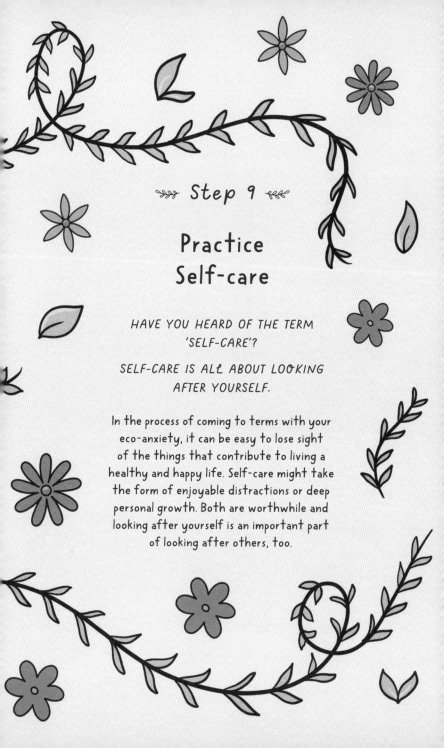

✦✦✦ Step 9 ✦✦✦

Practice
Self-care

HAVE YOU HEARD OF THE TERM 'SELF-CARE'?

SELF-CARE IS ALL ABOUT LOOKING AFTER YOURSELF.

In the process of coming to terms with your eco-anxiety, it can be easy to lose sight of the things that contribute to living a healthy and happy life. Self-care might take the form of enjoyable distractions or deep personal growth. Both are worthwhile and looking after yourself is an important part of looking after others, too.

Have you ever heard the phrase, 'you can't pour from an empty cup'?

This saying means that in order for us as humans to effectively take care of others, we must first take care of ourselves. It's like when you're on an aeroplane and hear the flight attendants say, "In the case of an emergency, for parents travelling with small children it's important that you put on your own oxygen mask first." They have to say this because this is the last thing most parents would ever think of doing. But it's vital that they get their own oxygen masks on quickly - because without oxygen they won't be physically capable of taking care of others. The reason I'm using this flight analogy is because when you become anxious about the state of the world it's easy to forget that you too are an important and precious part of it. Not only that, but we need you at your best so you can become part of the solution.

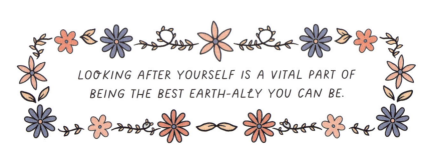

LOOKING AFTER YOURSELF IS A VITAL PART OF BEING THE BEST EARTH-ALLY YOU CAN BE.

If you're drained of hope and energy, or if you don't like yourself very much, it can be tempting to give up - and I think we're all agreed that this isn't a good idea. So, not only is it important to be real and let yourself feel the sadness, it's also important to top yourself up with happiness and energy - just like a planet-friendly refillable jar. **You may be asking at this point, is it even possible to feel good in the middle of a crisis? I'm here to tell you: yes, it is.**

A couple of years ago I spoke to a doctor who works in Tasmania, a part of Australia that was particularly affected by bushfires in 2020. Not only were her patients stressed about climate change, so was she. She told me the only way she could cope was to practice 'functional denial'. This might sound a bit odd - isn't denial the thing we're meant to be fighting against? What she meant was that she had to switch off from the problem on a regular basis, otherwise she'd be overwhelmed. If she wanted to keep looking after her patients, she had to do things that helped her temporarily to forget what was going on.

Rather than thinking of it as completely pushing the problem out of your mind, maybe it's more helpful to imagine changing your focus. If you look closely at the palm of your hand, the rest of your surroundings goes fuzzy. You know they're still there, but you lose sight of everything else and get lost in the lines, the lumps and bumps and maybe the way the light makes the skin shiny in places. It can be useful to shift your focus away from life's problems once in a while. The most important thing you need to know about the distraction, or 'functional denial', part of self-care is that it's for you, so only you have to like it.

It's all very well for people to tell you to meditate or do yoga, but what if you think that sounds a bit boring? Maybe you're the sort of person who prefers jumping on a trampoline or practicing ballet. Or perhaps you like doing origami, or trying to rap faster than Dizzee Rascal. You could be into literally anything! That's one of the things that's so brilliant about people - we're all different.

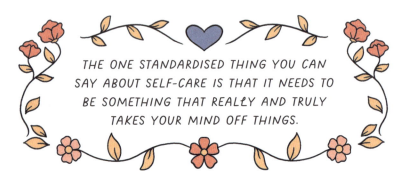

THE ONE STANDARDISED THING YOU CAN SAY ABOUT SELF-CARE IS THAT IT NEEDS TO BE SOMETHING THAT REALLY AND TRULY TAKES YOUR MIND OFF THINGS.

Who knew that this could be a crucial part of caring for the Earth? But it can! Nothing is too trivial or odd. It just has to work for you.

It probably goes without saying that some of the things we like might be bad for the planet, so these obviously aren't going to work as self-care activities. When we talk about functional denial, we mean a kind of temporary denial that helps to keep us functioning, but it also has to be 'functional' in relation to the environment. Buying some fast fashion to take your mind off the emergency, for instance, would be better off being called 'dysfunctional denial'. And that's definitely no way to help yourself feel better!

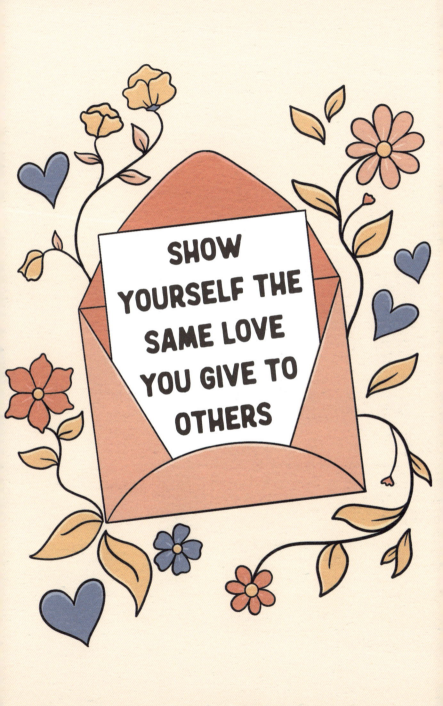

Self-care activities

Here are some self-care activites for very different types of people. I know you're completely unique, and not a 'type' at all, but at least this might give you some ideas to start off with. Maybe you're even a little bit of each - in which case mix it up!

SELF-CARE FOR EXTROVERTS

Talk to a friend. Talk to ten friends. Throw a party. Put on a funny outfit or even get a wild haircut so that everyone talks to you!

SELF-CARE FOR INTROVERTS

Read a book. Listen to a podcast. Build a den at home. Create artwork. Talk to a friend (just maybe not ten at once). Introverts have friends, too!

SELF-CARE FOR SPORTY TYPES

Go for a walk, run, swim or bike ride. Or maybe all four! See how many skips you can do with a skipping rope. You could invent a way of measuring how high you can jump.

SELF-CARE FOR RELAXED TYPES

Sleep loads. Have a bubble bath. Lie on the carpet and stare at the ceiling. Watch a movie you liked when you were little, even if you've seen it a hundred times - or especially if you've seen it a hundred times!

SELF-CARE FOR CLEVER TYPES

Learn to write and say a few words in Sanskrit. Try to understand what Einstein was on about. Study Greek myths. Find out what makes water wet.

Ways to cultivate your character

1 FRIENDLINESS

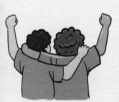

One of the most terrifying myths about the future is that resources will become so scarce that humans will turn against one another in a battle for survival. But there is another possible future where people help each other when the going gets tough. We can start that future now.

2 CURIOSITY

Curious people ask good questions and seek out good answers. In other words, they are problem-solvers and are open to new worlds and possibilities. Curiosity is also a friendly character trait as it involves being interested in the thoughts of others.

3 COURAGE

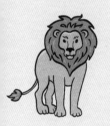

It goes without saying that moving into an uncertain future requires a huge amount of courage. A bit like 'functional denial', courage can involve temporarily pushing certain ideas out of your mind so you can do what needs to be done. Courage and hope go very well together: courage requires hope and hope requires courage.

4 GRATITUDE

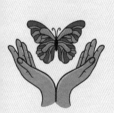

We live on a most extraordinary planet. And we live on it at a time where we are well-placed to understand its extraordinariness scientifically as well as intuitively. We know how incredible it is that our ecosystems produce food and water. Be glad to be alive.

5 CALM

Calm is perhaps the hardest quality to cultivate, but it rubs off on other people too, so it's worthwhile thinking about how to let go of your worries and just **BE** once in a while.

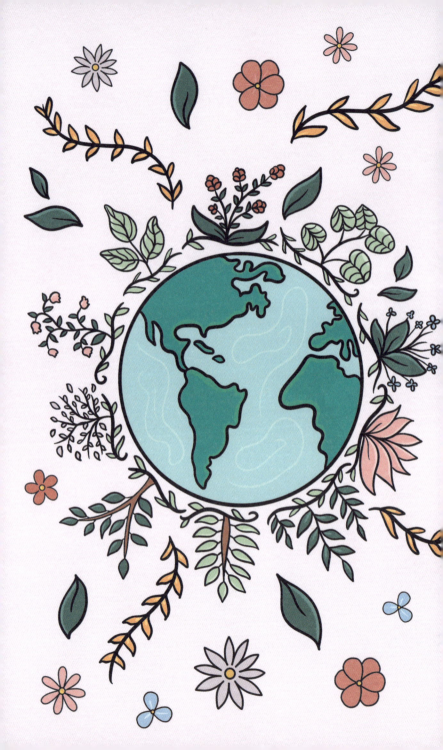

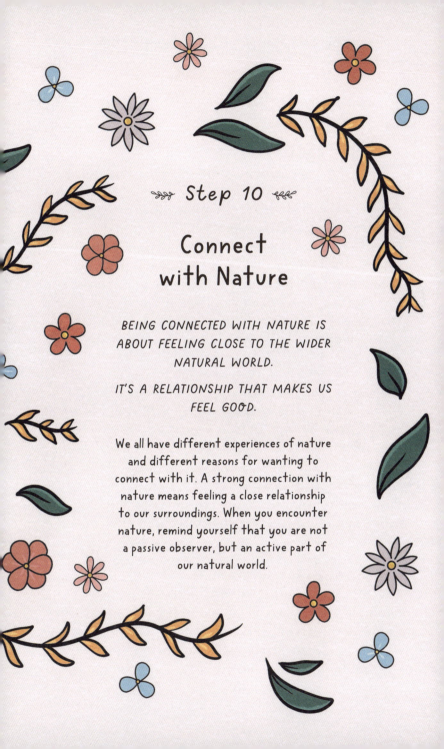

~~~ Step 10 ~~~

Connect
with Nature

*BEING CONNECTED WITH NATURE IS
ABOUT FEELING CLOSE TO THE WIDER
NATURAL WORLD.*

*IT'S A RELATIONSHIP THAT MAKES US
FEEL GOOD.*

We all have different experiences of nature
and different reasons for wanting to
connect with it. A strong connection with
nature means feeling a close relationship
to our surroundings. When you encounter
nature, remind yourself that you are not
a passive observer, but an active part of
our natural world.

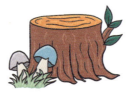

Nature has always been all around us.

Around two hundred and fifty years ago, during a time known as the Industrial Revolution (when people in Britain, Europe and America began to rely much more heavily on the use of machines and chemicals), people were in conflict about the purpose of nature. Was it a terrible, destructive force that needed to be controlled and tamed? Or was it a state of bliss that we needed to make our way back to? You could say, well, obviously the second one, but it turns out not to be so simple.

One of the problems with thinking of nature as intrinsically charming and good was that maybe it only looked that way to certain people because they were seeing it through the lens of 'culture'. It was all very well for rich, white industrialists to sit in their stately homes, eating buttered crumpets made from the products of industrial agriculture and moan about being disconnected from the natural world. But what if that was just their wealthy, white privilege speaking? Maybe they only liked nature on the condition that other people were taking care of it for them. (And by 'taking care' I mean 'destroying'.)

This unfortunate history has left its mark on those who live in industrial societies, so much so that the only flower species some people see are the ones being sold in the supermarket. These days, even if you live right in the middle of the countryside your relationship with nature is likely to be affected by industrialisation. So where should you go to look for it?

Can you find nature in an inner-city park? A zoo? The rolling fields of a green and pleasant, yet intensively farmed countryside? Or do you have to go to an ancient forest, or perhaps to the bottom of the ocean? And what will you do when you get there? Take a photo? Or wander about in dream-like awe, stroking every leaf and waving at every unsuspecting creature?

Perhaps the main thing we need to truly understand about nature is that it's not 'over there' for us to go and visit; it's everywhere. Those of us who live in big cities might not feel like we encounter much wild foliage in our day-to-day lives, but even the air around us is part of the natural world. It moves and blows and dissipates, and if we fill it with toxic fumes these will pollute the atmosphere. Even in the busiest city you can find animals in the early morning before the day's bustle begins. From bugs and birds to rabbits and rats, nature can be found in every nook and cranny. Even the weeds that grow up through our pavements, or the bushes that line our streets, are a part of nature.

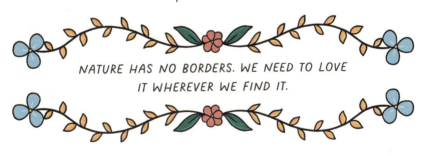

NATURE HAS NO BORDERS. WE NEED TO LOVE IT WHEREVER WE FIND IT.

Nature is really good for us too. Research suggests that people with a greater connection to nature are more likely to be happier and behave positively towards the environment.

But connecting with nature doesn't mean having a special, isolated experience and then going back to your life. Nor does it have to mean living in a self-sufficient community. It means appreciating the world in its enormity and understanding that it forms one gigantic, staggering ecosystem.

If you are lucky enough to have seen a mountain range, jungle or wild beach then you will know that being in unspoiled nature affects the way you think. It's so sublime and impressive it can make your own worries seem tiny. It's exciting to see rock formations, giant plants, or seals diving in the waves. Nature gives us so much to occupy our minds with - it's limitlessly fascinating and beautiful. Many towns and cities contain wonderful botanical gardens, tended according to natural principles, where you can really feel nature at work. Even in densely populated areas you can often find densely overgrown railway sidings or thriving patches of lush, untended foliage. If you look for nature in an open-minded way you will find it, and you won't have to go very far.

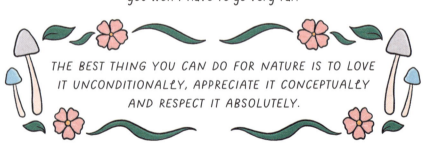

THE BEST THING YOU CAN DO FOR NATURE IS TO LOVE IT UNCONDITIONALLY, APPRECIATE IT CONCEPTUALLY AND RESPECT IT ABSOLUTELY.

You can love nature whoever and wherever you are. You don't need money, you don't need transport, you don't need permission. All you need is compassion, understanding and a big, big heart.

NATURE IS NOT
A PLACE TO VISIT.

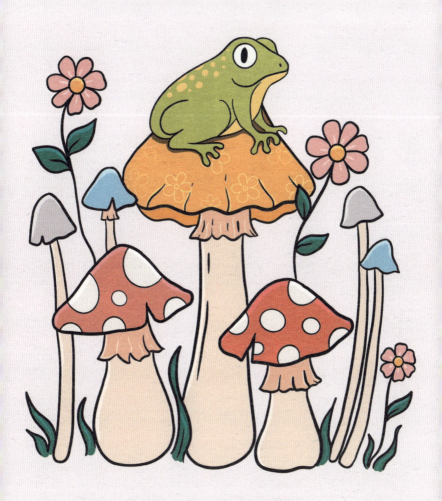

IT IS HOME.

Ways to connect with nature

1 DISCOVER PLANTS ON YOUR DOORSTEP

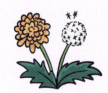

All of nature is a marvel. It's every bit as incredible to see a buddleia or a dandelion bursting though concrete as it is to see a jungle. Dandelions especially are popular with pollinators. If you have a garden, leave your dandelions alone - even if they're right in the middle of your lawn!

2 LOOK OUT FOR EVERY CRITTER

Ecosystems don't run on cuteness. Every living creature is important and even the most dangerous, stinky or stingy animal has its place in the world. Just like wasps - not only are they great pollinators but they prey on greenfly and other insects that might otherwise destroy our crops.

3 LEARN ABOUT HUMAN HISTORY

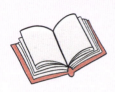

If we're going to have a future where we don't repeat the mistakes of our past, we need to have a good understanding of our history. Learn what you can about industrialisation and globalisation and see how they have shaped the world we live in today.

4 GET INTERESTED IN THE WEATHER

It's not only plants and animals that will determine our survival, but weather too. Instead of just listening to the weather report on the news, ask yourself what weather is. Why does the wind blow, the rain fall, the fog lift? All weather can be beautiful!

5 THINK ABOUT SPACE

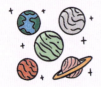

Sometimes life on Earth can seem completely overwhelming. When things down here are really getting to you it can be such a relief to think about the universe. After all, in the grand scheme of things the whole universe is 'nature'.

Engaging with your senses

The Japanese have a term, 'shinrin yoku', which translates as 'forest bathing'. It means using all your senses to engage with nature in order to feel its calming, therapeutic benefits. It doesn't even need to be in a forest, just the nearest and best bit of nature you can find.

SMELL

Enjoy the subtle smells of plants. It's not only roses and lavender that smell wonderful, even humble grass or damp leaves have a delicious, soothing aroma.

TOUCH

Notice the different textures of plants. Some are stiff and shiny while others are soft and hairy. Maybe lie on the ground and feel the solidity of the earth beneath you. Stroke some bark, or even just hug the whole tree.

LOOK

Gaze up through the leaves to the sky. Perhaps take a close-up photograph showing the incredible detail in a tiny part of nature. You could be the only person who's ever focussed on that little section of the universe.

TASTE

If you're fortunate enough to have a friend or family member with a good knowledge of edible wild plants, ask them to take you foraging. Perhaps you will find wild garlic, or nettles to make into tea.

LISTEN

Open your ears to the sounds of birds and insects, or the air moving through the leaves. No composer can compete with the natural sounds of the world, and no technology can capture the immersive surround-sound of life as it unfolds around you.

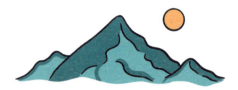

We've been on quite a journey together throughout this book.

I feel privileged to have been given a space to put down some thoughts. I hope some of my thoughts have been helpful. They're not even solely *my* thoughts, really. They're a mixture of lots of people's thoughts all arranged together in one place. Take a moment to digest and acknowledge how you're feeling. When you turn the page, you'll find ideas on ways to express what eco-anxiety means to you.

I love to express my feelings through writing. When I wrote my first climate-related book thirty years ago, most of us thought that the environmental changes we feared were at least a few generations away. One of the biggest shocks has been how fast small changes in planetary temperature make a huge difference to both weather systems and ecosystems.

I feel so sorry that my generation didn't do nearly enough. In a sense, climate change is both expected and unexpected. We saw it coming and we didn't. Even now, we can't predict exactly how it's going to unfold. But it seems that you and I are likely to witness extraordinary events that will change the ways we think about the world and how we inhabit it. People all over the world are fighting hard to bring about changes that need to be made, and I know you will be part of that battle. But always remember that our strongest force is love. With all of our love, and the actions that spring from it, the future is bright.

Before you sit down to put pen to paper, or finger to keyboard, have a look back at some of the things you've learned. Maybe the main thing is never to feel alone with your fears. Since I've been researching the field of eco-anxiety, the thing I've probably read most often is that it helps to talk to other people about it. Sometimes even I find myself thinking, 'What's the point?' But then I find myself having a really good chat with a friend (or sometimes a stranger) and it actually turns out to be true. **Talking about the climate emergency really, truly helps.** Sometimes it just helps you, sometimes it also helps the other person and, if enough of us do it, it can also help the planet.

Then there's all the other stuff, like not being afraid to have feelings. Or trying not to let the size of the problem get on top of you. Or taking care of yourself and fostering your resilience. And above all, always letting your love for the planet guide your actions. There is a wonderful climate change campaigner called Aubrey Meyer whose work was nominated for the Nobel Peace Prize in 2008. He says we should be like musicians and start playing together harmoniously.

We need to think like an orchestra with all its different instruments: if enough of us start to play in tune and in time we can make extraordinary things happen.

Creativity is a vital part of life. Art, music and poetry aren't just a luxury for times when everything else is going well. We need to know we can express ourselves at all times and in all situations. People have written beautiful poems on battlefields, in refugee camps, or while they were chronically ill. **Art never stops.**

Here are some ways to give form to your thoughts and feelings about climate change:

WRITE A POEM

Decide whether you want it to rhyme or not. It can be long or short, sad or celebratory. You could choose a plant or an animal as a theme, or just make it about your feelings. It could even be a scientific poem!

WRITE A STORY

Your story can be as imaginative or as factual as you like. It could be more like a fairy tale or a newspaper article. Of course, it can be sad or scary, but it could also be funny. Sometimes the most serious situations can be greatly improved by a good joke.

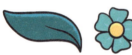

WRITE A SONG

It would be good if pop stars could be a bit more vocal about the climate. It's strange that so few of them are. Maybe what the world needs is a massive hit record about the climate emergency. Written by you – no pressure!

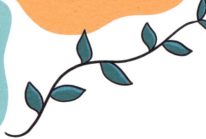

WRITE A JOURNAL

Keeping a journal is a great way to organise your thoughts and feelings. You can say whatever you like without worrying about what anyone else will think. Having said that, if you choose to write a story or song further down the line, it can be a really useful source of ideas.

WRITE A LETTER

It could be to a friend or someone you admire. Perhaps it could be a thank you letter for something they've done for the climate. You could get other people to sign it with you.

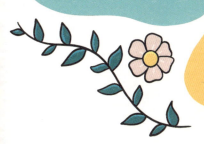

To say farewell, I've written a haiku just for you. If you didn't know already, a haiku is a Japanese poem of seventeen syllables, in three lines of five, seven and five. They traditionally evoke images of the natural world. Mine's titled *Leaves* – I hope you enjoy it and close this book feeling inspired to write your own.

 Leaves

I HEARD A RUSTLE.

THE FUTURE WAS WHISPERING,

'PLEASE COME AND JOIN ME'.

ACTIVISM – the actions people take to make the changes they want to see in the world.

AGENCY – the ability to take action or choose what action to take.

CARBON-NEUTRAL – not increasing the overall amount of carbon dioxide in the earth's atmosphere.

CATASTROPHISE – to imagine the worst possible outcome.

CLIMATE CHANGE – changes in the Earth's climate, especially the gradual rise in temperature caused by high levels of carbon dioxide.

CLIMATE DENIAL – refusing to accept that climate change is happening.

COGNITIVE DISSONANCE – anxiety that results from simultaneously holding contradictory attitudes or beliefs.

COLLECTIVE ACTION – action taken together by a group of people who aim to achieve a common objective.

CONTRADICTION – a situation where two or more ideas are in opposition to one another.

COPING MECHANISM – something a person does to deal with a difficult situation.

DEFEATIST – someone who thinks or talks in a way that suggests that they expect to be unsuccessful.

ECO-ANXIETY – a state of distress caused by concern about damage to the environment.

ECOLOGICAL THOUGHT – the idea of interconnectedness.

ECOSYSTEM – all the plants and animals that live in a particular area together with the complex relationship that exists between them and their environment.

EMISSION – a substance that is produced and sent out into the air. Some are harmful to the environment, especially carbon dioxide or methane.

ENVIRONMENTALIST – a person who protects the environment.

EXTROVERT – a socially confident person.

FAST FASHION – the reproduction of clothes at high speed and low cost. These clothes are often worn once and then thrown away.

FLEXITARIANISM – a diet centered on plant foods with the occasional inclusion of meat or fish.

FORAGING – finding food by hunting, fishing or gathering.

FOSSIL FUEL – fuel such as coal or oil that is formed from the decayed remains of plants or animals.

GLOBALISATION – the process by which the world is becoming interconnected because of increased trade and cultural exchange.

🍄 GLOSSARY 🍄

GLOBAL NORTH – the richest and most industrialised countries, which are mainly in the northern part of the world.

INDUSTRIALISATION – the shift away from agriculture towards manufactured goods, which are often produced by machines.

INNER CRITIC – a negative internal voice.

JARGON – special words and phrases that are used by particular groups of people, especially in their work.

MISINFORMATION – the spreading of false ideas.

OPTIMISM – the tendency to see the good side of things or to expect the best in any situation.

OVERFISHING – catching too many fish in an area of the sea, so that there are not many fish left there.

PARASYMPATHETIC – nervous system a network of nerves that relaxes your body after periods of stress or danger.

PESSIMISM – the tendency to see the bad side of things or to expect the worst in any situation.

PSYCHOTHERAPIST – a person who treats mental suffering by psychological rather than medical means.

RENEWABLE ENERGY – energy produced from sources like the sun and wind that are naturally replenished and do not run out.

RESILIENCE – the ability to bounce back from difficulties.

REWILDING – the practice of returning areas of land to a wild state, including the reintroduction of animal species that are no longer naturally found there.

RUMINATION – obsessive repetition of thoughts.

SAFE SPACE – a place where people can openly discuss their thoughts.

SELF-CARE – the practice of looking after one's own wellbeing

SPECIES – a set of animals or plants in which the members have similar characteristics to each other and can breed with each other.

SUSTAINABLE – causing little or no damage to the environment and therefore able to continue for a long time.

SYMPATHETIC NERVOUS SYSTEM – a network of nerves that helps your body activate its 'fight-or-flight' response.

TIPPING POINT – the point at which a series of small changes or incidents becomes significant enough to cause a larger, more important change.

VALIDATION – recognition or affirmation that a person or their feelings or opinions are valid or worthwhile.

Find out more about how to better understand the climate crisis and deal with eco-anxiety with the help of an adult.

BOOKS

Generation Green by Linda Sivertsen

How You Can Save the Planet by Hendrikus van Hensbergen

No One is Too Small to Make a Difference by Greta Thunberg

We Have a Dream by Mya-Rose Craig and Sabrena Khadija

PODCASTS

BBC Earth Kids
Celebrating nature, science and the human race.

Climate Crisis Conversations
Thoughtful conversations between climate psychologists about the climate crisis. These two episodes are child-friendly:

'Episode 5: Deep Questioning: Navigating youth at a time of climate change'

'Episode 13: From Anxiety to Agency: Stepping up, rather than shutting down, in the face of the climate change crisis'

WEBSITES

BBC Children in Need
Wellbeing advice and resources for eco-anxiety.

www.bbcchildreninneed.co.uk/ changing-lives/understanding- the-climate-crisis-and-eco-anxiety

Force of Nature
A website which empowers young people to turn their eco-anxiety into agency.

www.forceofnature.xyz

Greenpeace
A movement of people passionate about protecting the natural world.

www.greenpeace.org.uk

Young Upstart
A hub of information for young people working together and empowering each other to save the planet.

www.ecoanxiety.com